Natural Healing
in Gynaecology

Rina Nissim was born in Jerusalem, although
she is now a Swiss national. Completing her
nursing training in 1975, she was a founder
member in 1978 of Dispensaire des Femmes, a
women's health centre collective, operating
from Geneva. She has been active in the
women's movement since 1972. She has experience of working with women and health groups
in the USA, Central America and India. *Natural
Healing in Gynaecology* has been published in
French, German, Italian, Spanish, Dutch,
Serbo-Croatian and Portuguese editions.

Natural Healing in Gynaecology

A Manual for Women

Rina Nissim

Translated from the French by
Roxanne Claire

An Imprint of HarperCollinsPublishers

For Dolly

Pandora
An Imprint of HarperCollins*Publishers*
77–85 Fulham Palace Road,
Hammersmith, London W6 8JB
1160 Battery Sreet
San Francisco, California 94111–1213

First published in English by Pandora Press
in association with Methuen, Inc., New York, 1986
This edition 1996
Originally published in French as *Mamamélis*
by Editions Dispensaire des Femmes, Geneva, 1984
3 5 7 9 10 8 6 4 2

© Editions Dispensaire des Femmes 1984
Translation © Rina Nissim 1986, 1996

Rina Nissim asserts the moral right to
be identified as the author of this work

A catalogue record for this book
is available from the British Library

ISBN 0 04 4409591

Printed and bound in Great Britain by
Caledonian International Book Manufacturing Ltd, Glasgow

Contents

* An asterisk indicates that a word is to be found in the Definitions on pages 204–10.
† A dagger indicates a drug brand name.
aa = in equal quantity   qsp = to arrive at a quantity of

Acknowledgements

This manual is largely inspired by the French phytotherapists H. Leclerc, J. Valnet, M. Tétau and C. Bergeret and M. Girault, by the Swiss herbalist de Vantery and a Swiss doctor, Dr Catherine Kousmine, and by several American and Chinese authors.

The application of their methods to gynaecology has been possible only thanks to the users[4] of the Women's Health Center, to their interest in 'new' methods, and to their confidence and their patience in the 'early days'.

Natural Healing in Gynaecology is dedicated to the women and health movement, and to all women everywhere!

---

[4] Translator's note: In keeping with the self-help philosophy, the women who come to the Women's Health Center are not referred to as 'patients', but 'users' (*usagères*).

Introduction

The self-help movement

Since its beginning more than fifteen years ago, the women and health movement has grown enormously. It is today an international phenomenon[1] – attesting both to women's role as health care providers and to the power inherent in understanding one's own body and its care.

The self-help movement grew out of women's realization of how we have been dispossessed of an immense knowledge (and thus power) by (male) doctors. Ever since witches ('wise women') skilled in the use of herbs and other remedies[2] were burned for knowing too much, women have been confined to subordinate roles as health care providers – nurses, pharmacy aides, etc. – while as health care seekers, they are treated as passive consumers. Obstetrics and Gynaecology is virtually a caricature of this loss of control. Labour room chairs are designed for the comfort of the attending physician, for example, not that of the woman in labour. The field of gynaecology is in fact almost entirely dominated by men, who have neither uterus

[1] See reports of the International Women and Health Conferences so far. Available from EFI (International Women's Space for documentation and solidarity), 2 rue de la Tannerie, 1227 Carouge, Geneva, Switzerland, and the Women's Global Network on Reproductive Rights Nieuwe Zijds Voorburgwal 32, 1012 RZ Amsterdam, The Netherlands, respectively.

[2] See *Witches, Midwives and Nurses*, Barbara Ehrenreich and Deirdre English, Glass Mountain Pamphlets, Oyster Bay, New York, 1973.

1

nor vagina and who have none the less become the new scholars of the female genital organs and their medicine.

But the self-help goal of putting information and control into the hands of women has yet deeper ramifications. In developing the kind of health care that meets women's needs, the self-help movement uses a *model of health care* which differs from that of modern western medicine, one which borrows extensively from the approach of natural healing.

One difference is in the concepts themselves of illness, health and health care. For modern western medicine, disease is caused by germs, bacteria and viruses, and health care consists of combatting enemy microbes with chemicals,[3] and interrupting the course of the disease. The natural healing approach, on the other hand, is a *holistic* one which recognizes the emotional, social and environmental factors in disease, and which treats the person as a whole being. Moreover, symptoms (disease) are regarded as an expression of the body's attempts to return to a certain equilibrium. Treatment of these symptoms, then, lies in helping the system concerned to do its work. For example, fasting or eating lightly when you have a fever helps the body by allowing it to focus on ridding itself of toxins already present, and not overburdening it further. Natural healing is also a more *preventive*, or health oriented, style of medicine, stressing how one stays in good health – for example, through diet – rather than focusing solely on treating each illness as it occurs.

Another difference lies in modern western medicine's *profit orientation*. In addition to spawning the pharmaceutical industry (not a few of whose products are – although expensive – ineffective if not downright dangerous), this means quality health care is sometimes available only to those who can afford to pay – and pay dearly – for it.

In contrast to the passive consumerism encouraged by modern medicine, and the information-for-sale (to be jealously guarded) attitude of modern medical practitioners, self-help seeks to encourage *autonomy* through *information sharing*.

---

[3] *Our Bodies, Ourselves*, Boston Women's Health Book Collective.

ﾞﾞ

Hazardous to your health

Modern western medicine's approach to gynaecology, then, is characterized by treatments which suppress symptoms without treating causes, and an unchecked use of synthetic hormones for a wide range of indications, from painful periods to acne to menopause. Consequences of such treatment can be serious: cardio-vascular diseases, cancer, tumours – not to mention the effect on the delicate hormone system! Clearly, modern western medicine, especially for women, ought to be labelled: 'Caution. May be hazardous to your health.'

ﾞﾞ

Alternatives

Alternatives are available in a growing number of women-run women's health clinics. The Women's Health Center is one such clinic. Collectively run, the Health Center has offered standard and alternative gynaecological care to the women of Geneva, Switzerland, since 1978. However, the Health Center is but one example of women-controlled health care, which is not limited to Europe and North America. This approach to health care, particularly when done in a group setting with group discussion, is appropriate for all women, including those in less economically privileged classes or countries. In addition, the therapeutic methods used in self-help, since they are based on what the Earth gives us in the form of locally available herbs, are applicable everywhere.

༃

About this book

Natural Healing in Gynaecology was written to describe the use of herbs, trace-elements and diet in ensuring the proper functioning of the body and in the treatment of gynaecological disorders. It is intended as a tool for health care workers interested in natural healing and in alternatives to modern western medicine.

At the same time, as a product of the self-help movement, this manual is equally intended for women seeking to deepen their knowledge of their own bodies and their health care.

The manual is divided into four parts. The first section covers disorders related to the menstrual cycle (Chapters 1–5); the second, infections (Chapters 6–12); the third, tumours (Chapters 13 and 14); and the fourth, diet and AIDS (Chapter 15 and 16). Each chapter includes a short explanation of the disorders and their possible origins, a brief description of what modern western medicine proposes in the way of treatment, and finally, the possible alternatives, with an emphasis on the use of herbs. Definitions, the principles of using tinctures and essential oils, a rapid description of diatheses in the use of trace-elements, and key references and useful addresses are to be found at the back of the book.

༃

A note on the use of herbs

As you will discover, herbal preparations can take a variety of forms. *Infusions** are a gentle yet effective way of keeping in good health. There may be situations, however, when you will find it necessary to use preparations whose active principles are more concentrated: *tinctures**, *essential oils**, *glycerine macerates**, and other remedies.

You will notice that several herbs may be mentioned for any

one specific disorder. Although most phytotherapists (herbalists) make associations between four and seven herbs, i.e. combine herbs together in a single treatment, it is not necessary to take all those mentioned. What is important is each herb's effect on *you*. Obviously, the most rigorous approach would be to try one herb at a time, in order to observe its effect.

Treating yourself, then, means observing your strengths, weaknesses, and illnesses, and requires a knowledge of herbs. This knowledge is acquired over time as you refer to works on phytotherapy (herbalism) describing the various herbs and determine, according to the different properties and indications of each one (and, eventually, your experience with them), which ones 'fit' you best.

It should be pointed out, however, that for the woman who seeks to treat herself, many of the methods described in these chapters will, alone, not suffice for curing certain illnesses. In such cases, this manual is more of a guide to what can be done, and is to be used with the aid of a health care worker.

In determining dosage, you will want to keep in mind that the doses mentioned here are averages. To tailor them to your needs, your weight and diet have to be taken into consideration. Those of you with 'clean diets', who do not smoke, will respond to smaller doses than those of you with heavy diets or who smoke.

This manual has its limitations. It was not possible to include information on acupuncture and homoeopathy as true 'ground' medicines, that is to say, an approach to health care which aims to modify tendencies to certain illnesses. Nor does this manual go into enough detail on the relationship of physical symptoms to the social, economic and psychological conditions of each woman's life. Each of these topics could fill several volumes. It is hoped, however, that the book will be but one part – to be followed by many others – of the reconstruction of a medicine for women, by women.

✌ **Brief Overview** ✌

Hormones and the Menstrual Cycle

Oestrogen is principally se-
creted by the ovaries (and the placenta during pregnancy).
Oestrogen levels peak twice during the menstrual cycle: just
before ovulation and in the middle of the second phase, when
the yellow body in the ovary is at its peak.

Oestrogen is responsible for developing and maintaining
the female sexual organs and for generally aiding in the
growth of tissue. It stimulates cellular division, especially in
the base layers of the mucous membrane of the mouth, the
skin, the nose, the urethra, the vagina, and the mammary
glands. It also contributes to the calcification of bones.
Oestrogen is responsible for the retention of water and salt,
hence weight gain. It makes the secretion of the sebaceous
glands more fluid, thus inhibiting the formation of acne (in
contrast to testosterone). Finally, its presence is accompanied
by a lowering of cholesterol in the blood and may inhibit the
formation of arteriosclerosis.

✌

Progesterone

Progesterone, formerly called luteum, is secreted by the
ovarian yellow body. Its role is to transform the mucous
membrane, overly developed by oestrogens, to render it more

welcoming to a possible fertilized ovum and more favourable to the development of the egg. It also makes pregnancy possible by inhibiting contractions and the tonus of the uterine muscle.

An excess of progesterone increases the appetite, contributes to weight gain, and causes fatigue, depression, diminution of libido, and acne.

This is a very brief résumé of the physiology of the menstrual cycle. For more information, see References (pages 219–22).

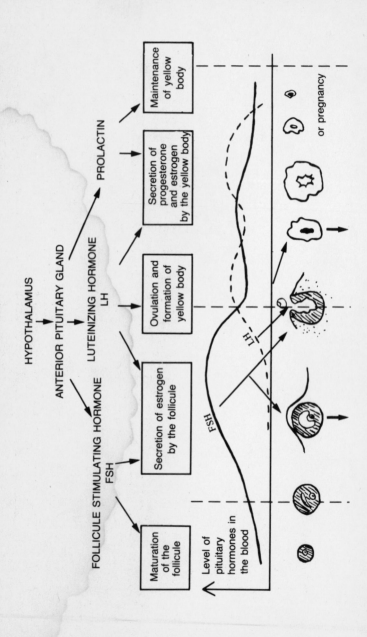

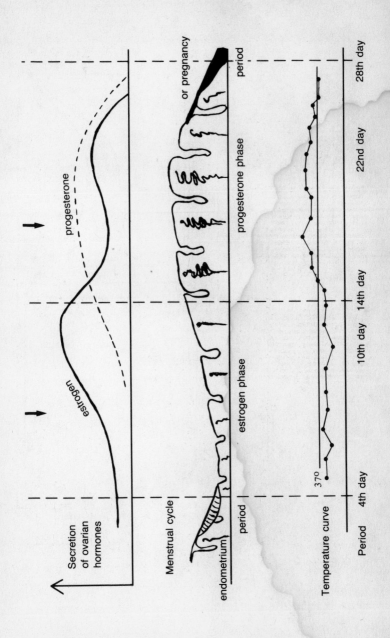

In more detail, or to better demonstrate the hormonal inter-play at the moment of ovulation:

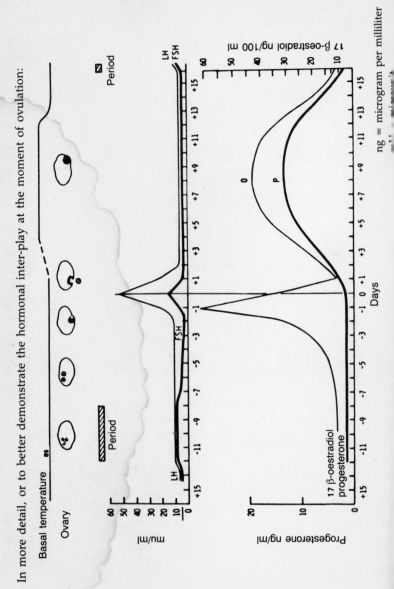

ng = microgram per milliliter

Disagreeable Signs Before Periods and at Ovulation

What a task to begin with such a difficult chapter! But as these are the complaints which are the most benign, the most frequent and the least taken into consideration by gynaecologists, let's plunge in.

The many disagreeable signs a woman can feel at the approach of her period or ovulation do not appear to have anything in common. The symptoms which we generally group under the name 'pre-menstrual syndrome' (PMS), can be diverse: sudden changes of character, desire for sweets, sleep difficulties, congestion (hard and sensitive breasts), bloated abdomen, constipation with accompanying risk of haemorrhoids caused by straining, water retention, weight gain, possible oedema, gall bladder problems with difficulty in evacuating bile, headaches, nausea, vomiting, cystitis, unusually abundant vaginal secretions, asthma, hives, herpes, acne, beginnings of a sore throat, colds, backache, looseness of ligaments which can mean repeated sprains . . . (whew!).

These symptoms are all related to an over-sensitization to sex hormones, a sort of self-poisoning.

Folliculine, or the oestrogen hormone secreted by the ovary, is responsible for the proliferation of uterine mucous membrane before ovulation. It is responsible, too, for the appearance of the female secondary sex characteristics. An over-secretion of this hormone results in hyperfolliculinemia or hyperoestrogenemia.

There are two possible explanations for this hypersecretion.

It may be due to an 'error' of FSH (follicule stimulating hormone, which is secreted by the pituitary gland), or it may be the result of an insufficiency of progesterone. This latter hypothesis is receiving more and more attention in medical circles, particularly in the United States where studies on progesterone insufficiency have been conducted on prisoners (!) and pre-menstrual tension has even been invoked as an attenuating circumstance in criminal trials!

Another factor involved is the *liver*. Where the liver is already overburdened by the responsibility of breaking down hormones and other 'toxins' (such as sugar, alcohol or drugs), it becomes less able to deal with peak levels of sex hormones (pre-menstrual and at ovulation). Thus, women become congested with their own hormones.

In addition, it is not unlikely that the continual use of hormones in the food industry also plays a role. This would explain the frequency of hyperfolliculinemia in gynaecological illnesses (as you will see in future chapters).

It is in fact the excess of oestrogens which causes the gastro-intestinal disorders, the water retention, and the excessive stimulation of oestrogen-sensitive tissues (such as the cervical mucus, the uterus and the breasts) which were described at the beginning of this chapter.

~

What does modern western medicine propose?

- preparations based on progesterone, which inhibit oestrogens and thus cause anovular cycles (ovulation does not occur) if they are taken during the entire cycle, or from the 15th to the 25th day of the cycle;
- sedatives and tranquillizers;
- psychotherapy;
- diuretics*.

ॐ

The alternatives

(a) *Dietary advice*

Reduce salt intake. This advice, also given to cardiac patients and the well-endowed, needs to be understood as the elimination of *refined table salt* which, because of processing, is unbalanced. Crude sea salt is less noxious; it is even indispensable to life. Meat and vegetables contain salt. Salt is involved in numerous organic processes, among others, the maintenance of an equilibrium of water in the body. To add salt (NaCl) during cooking and again at the table, however, is an abuse common in western cultures.

It might be mentioned here that in the struggle against water retention, it is not recommended to drink less. Water is a natural diuretic and the organs of elimination work better when the volume of circulating water is high.

Increase intake of potassium (K). Potassium is a cardiac and muscular tonic. It stimulates intestinal movements, intervenes in the regulation of adrenals and also plays a role in the balance of water in the body. Sodium is exchanged against potassium, so in the case of excess sodium, there is a loss of potassium. Potassium is found in: rice, wheat, potatoes, grapes, bananas, peanuts, pears, dates, cabbage, beans, hazelnuts, almonds and pollen.

Increase intake of vitamin B6. Vitamin B6 is found in green vegetables, soya, potatoes, egg yolk, pollen and yeasts. The necessary daily dose is 2 to 4 mg. Vitamin fans suggest taking 200 to 500 mg each day during the entire cycle (American style)!!

Take magnesium and calcium. The recommended daily allowance is 250 mg of magnesium per 125 mg of calcium. See chapter 2 on painful periods for the foods which contain Mg and Ca.

Increase intake of vitamin A, particularly where there is a problem of painful breasts at the end of the cycle. Vitamin A is found in: carrots, garlic, onions, tomatoes, spinach, peaches, berries, lentils, gooseberries, raspberries and mulberries, apricots, lemons, turnips, rose hips, grains, oleaginous fruits and vegetable oils. For a diet which is atoxic and full of vitamins, you should avoid constipation and tiring the liver with fried foods, cooked eggs, chocolate, alcohol . . . and should stimulate the gall bladder with black radish, artichokes, and olives as an aperitif. (Chapter 15 is dedicated entirely to diet.)

(b) *Herbs and other natural remedies*

Let's take a look at the herbs which can be useful in this situation.

To diminish hyperestronemia: the progesterone-like herbs (which imitate progesterone): tincture of chaste tree, lady's mantle, sarsaparilla and gromwell. This last herb is a diuretic and inhibitor of the pituitary gland. For this reason North Americans use it as a contraceptive. See also under amenorrhea, page 61.

The hormonal regulators: glycerine macerates or tincture of: raspberry, blackcurrant, rose hip and birch (betula pubens) for its excellent effect on breast tensions, while betula alba is used more as a diuretic. The hops (Humulus lupulus) and the oil of onager (Oenothera biennis)*, for its rich content of polyunsaturated fatty acids, can also be considered hormonal regulators.

Drainers and ground remedies (deep):

* magnesium in either capsule or trace-element form;
* hepato-vesicular drainer: tincture: boldo, combretum, black radish; European lindenwood, cypress, caraway, rosemary, thyme, pansy;
  Renal drainers: European linden, pansy, heather, uva ursi, rest-harrow;
* shave grass (key remineralizer, rich in silicum);
* pollen and honey.

Calming agents and tranquillizers:

* hawthorn, peony, sweet clover, black horehound, pasque flower, passion flower, valerian, white willow

- sleep disturbances: lithium in trace-element form, angelica, witch hazel, primrose, clove.

It is recommended to take the hormonal regulators such as raspberry, blackcurrant and rose hips in the first phase of the cycle, and the progesterone-like herbs in the second. Space doses of drainers throughout the cycle, taking special care against forgetfulness during the second phase.

The majority of these herbs will be covered in future chapters, but let's take a closer look at:

Cynorrhodon – Rose hip Fruit of sweet-brier, particularly rich in vitamins C, B, E, K, PP, A, and in tanin and pectin.

Properties: astringent, hemostatic, diuretic, depurative, anti-anaemia tonic, and vermifuge.

Indications: diarrhoea, white vaginal discharge, haemorrhage, urinary lithiasis, lack of vitamins, fatigue, spring cure, ascaris (intestinal parasitic worms).

Infusion of berries: 5 to 10 berries per cut, boil 2 minutes, then press through a cloth. Drink 3 to 4 cups per day.

(c) *Acupressure (massage of the points of acupuncture)*
A simple recommendation: stimulate the 4 large intestine, disperse the 6 spleen and pancreas.[1] For the sites of the points, useful for irregular periods, see page 34.

Stimulate: press deeply with the end of the fingers while vibrating the finger slightly and turning in a clockwise direction

Disperse: massage broadly the zone of the point in a counter-clockwise direction.

---

[1] these are names of acupuncture/acupressure points.

๙ 2 ๛

Painful Periods

Why and how do so many women experience such painful menstrual periods? Some women have a uterus which is very retroverted, that is, tipped toward the rectum rather than forward and toward the bladder (see diagram, page 209). Others have had a severe pelvic infection (infection of the uterus, Fallopian tubes, or peritoneum) and painful periods are a consequence. Still others have endometriosis, a gynaecological ailment with little-known causes, which is characterized by the appearance of tissue similar to the 'endometrium' (tissue which lines the uterine walls) outside the uterus, on the Fallopian tubes, on the peritoneum, and so on. These tissues bleed during periods and cause severe pain (see Chapter 12). However, many women who have retroverted uteruses or who have had a uterine infection do not have painful periods. In any case, these three possibilities account for only 20 per cent of the women who complain of painful periods.

This leaves us with 80 per cent of women whose primary or secondary dysmenorrhea is described as being due to hysteria, refusal of femininity, or masochistic character. Similarly, 'homosexuality and certain solitary sexual and other habits' (sic) are classed among the causes of secondary dysmenhorrhea (or the evident organic cause!) by Belaiche (see References). But let's leave the mazes of women-hating modern medicine.

Western and eastern medicines disagree on hygiene during

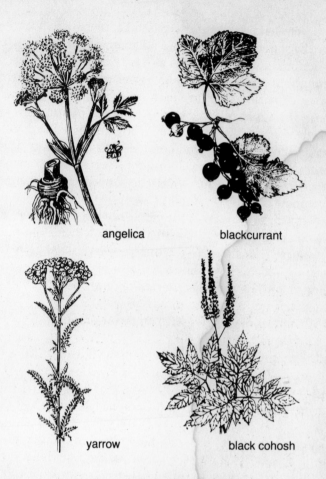

angelica   blackcurrant

yarrow   black cohosh

menstrual periods. American authors believe that women ought to maintain normal activities during periods; they ought even to be encouraged in sports. For the Chinese, on the other hand, periods are a time of least resistance for women; they should therefore be relieved of heavy tasks.

Indeed, it is a complex phenomenon which is taking place: the level of sex hormones falls, the mucus loosens, and uterine contractions empty the uterine cavity in a few days. Pain may be due to a spasm of the cervix with retention of menstrual fluid above the cervix. Clots may form which are even more painful to pass. It is possible too that a uterine contraction is experienced as painful because of pelvic congestion, because of a peri-uterine inflammation, or because of an associated constipation. It is also possible that pain felt most strongly in the lower back is associated with a retroverted uterus or with a back problem (at the lumbar or sacroilliac level) which is aggravated by the menstrual period.

Other factors which may be involved include the emotional significance, such as whether bleeding represents a failed attempt to conceive, the amount of stress in the woman's life situation, and the general attitude towards menstruation (as something dirty, for example).

Pain due to a spasm of the cervix ought to disappear with a pregnancy and especially with a vaginal delivery, but this can hardly be considered a treatment. Cervical dilation under local or general anaesthesia can also be done. Likewise the nerves may be surgically removed or destroyed . . . I will spare you the names of these methods.

What does modern western medicine propose?

- the suppression of ovulation, with the Pill;
- antispasmodics and analgesics;
- relaxation;
- supportive psychotherapy (occasionally).

Let's take a closer look at the proposed analgesics. The majority are based on aspirin, whose pain killing properties can be attributed to the caffeine (better to drink coffee!) or to the codeine. Three of the latest in the hormonal range in the United States are mefenamic acid (Ponstan†), naproxen (proxem†) and ibuprofen (Motrin†) inhibitors of prostaglandin, and frequently used to relieve arthritic pain. The side effects on the stomach are unfortunately similar to those of aspirin (burns, ulcers).

۶

The alternatives

(a) *Dietary advice*

Calcium, the most important mineral element in bones, also plays a role in the coagulation of the blood. It also has a part to play in maintaining an equilibrium in the nervous system and is necessary to the proper functioning of the sympathetic nervous system. This is the part of the nervous system which 'screams' during painful periods.

Calcium is found in wheat, oats, walnuts, hazelnuts, almonds, carrots, cabbage, spinach, caraway, potatoes, onions and turnips as well as in dairy products, cheeses and pollen. The daily requirement for calcium is between 0.5 and 2g and there is from 100 to 120mg in 100g of milk.

Clearly, the problem is not to find calcium, but to absorb it – for calcium is absorbed only in the presence of vitamins, A, C and D.

Magnesium is a factor in growth, cellular regeneration, psychological equilibrium and the vago-sympathetic system. It is also a hepatic drainer and an antiseptic. It is found in wheat, oats, corn, dates, spinach, potatoes, beets, and pollen, as well as in several fruits. The minimum daily requirement is 250mg.

Lack of magnesium in the diet is a result of human error: the excessive refining of grains in order to obtain white flour, and the refining of salt.

Carrots are rich in vitamins A, B and C, as well as in numerous minerals: iron, calcium, sodium, potassium and magnesium. The carrot, especially known as an intestinal regularizer, has numerous other properties including the capacity to render menstrual blood more liquid and periods less painful. Thus, a glass of freshly pressed carrot juice each morning of the week preceding the period can be recommended.

It is also recommended to avoid animal proteins (eggs, dairy products, meat, fish) the week before menstrual bleeding because they are more difficult to digest and more toxic than vegetable proteins (legumes, cereals, soya, sprouted grains, dried fruit). A day of fasting just before the menstrual period or the first day of the period can accelerate decongestion.

(b) *Other*

Among the other means which do not imply the use of any kind of medication, *heat* should be mentioned. A simple hot water bottle on the abdomen or lower back provides relief for many women. *Orgasm* provides complete and immediate relief but unfortunately may be followed by a new contraction of pain. Also to be mentioned are poultices of *sea salt*. Sea salt is heated and placed on the sacrum in an envelope of gauze or fine cloth.

Exercise: I can't restrain myself from presenting here in the second chapter a method which could in fact be presented in any of the chapters, since it is a set of yoga exercises specific to the functioning of the female genital organs. This method, perfected by Aviva Steiner (of Israel), stimulates the circulation of energy in the pelvic area, and in particular teaches a control of the pelvic muscles through exercises of contraction and relaxation. Aviva, a former yoga teacher, travelled in a number of different countries and learned the ancient dances and exercises which women have used for centuries to control the menstrual cycle. Actually a form of yoga, the exercises are rather demanding and need to be worked up to gradually. The series begins with exercises which help you to feel the muscles in the area. These are followed by three consecutive sequences of exercises done to lively music. The entire series takes an hour and a half. The principal movement consists of throwing the pelvis forward in a violent movement, while contracting the muscles in the area: buttocks, anus, vagina . . . The rapid repetition of this movement increases the circulation of the blood and directs it towards the uterus. It is not known exactly how it works, but the practice of these exercises before periods makes the periods not only painless but also shorter and less abundant. We will come back to these exercises in the next few chapters as they can be used in cases of irregular cycles, delayed periods, and so on.

(c) *The herbs*
  The analgesics
Yarrow (*Achillea millefolium*)
Part used: flower tops.
Properties: tonic, anti-spasmodic, utero-ovarian sedative, brings on periods, hemostatic, diuretic.
Indications: general fatigue, spasms, painful periods, menopausal complaints, absence of periods, circulatory complaints.
Infusion: 30g per litre, 3 cups per day.

Angelica (*Angelica archangelica*)
Parts used: seeds, roots.
Properties: stimulant, digestive tonic, anti-spasmodic, emmenagogue (brings on and regularizes periods), digestive.
Indications: fatigue, digestive atony, hepatic insufficiency, problems with periods.
Infusion: 40g or 1 fistful per litre, 1 cup after each meal.
Tincture: 20 to 30 drops before meals.

Lady's mantle (*Alchemilla vulgaris*)
Part used: entire plant.
Properties: astringent*, facilitates digestion, diuretic, decongestion agent of the organs (liver) and elective action on female organs, sedative.
Indications: painful or overly abundant periods, spasms, hepatic congestion, headaches, facilitates childbirth.
Decoction: 1 fistful per litre.
Tincture: 10 drops in a little water, 3 times a day.

Black cohosh (*Cimicifuga raremosa*)
Part used: whole plant, roots.
Properties: reflex moderator of nervous system, vascular anti-spasmodic, diuretic.
Indications: childbirth, neuralgia, hypertension, spasms, painful periods.
Decoction of the root: 1 teaspoon per cup, 3 cups per day.

This herb has a taste which is a little disgusting and it makes your head spin a little (some would say that it's 'giddying'), but not disagreeably so.

Blue cohosh (*Caulophyllum thalictroides*)
A decoction of the root (boiled for 10 minutes) is particularly indicated where pain results from *spasm of the cervix* (pain which can begin before the onset of bleeding) or by *delayed periods*. See too page 31.

Camomile
Part used: flowers.
Properties: anti-spasmodic, analgesic, gastric stimulant, stimulates the formation of leucocytes, emmenagogue.
Indications: migraines, difficult digestion, painful periods.
In external use: conjunctivitis and vulvar infections.
Infusion: 1 tablespoon per cup.
Tincture: 10 drops, twice a day.

And getting a little ahead of ourselves:

The hormonal regulators
Raspberry (*Rubus idaeus*)
Part used: leaf, bud.
Properties: astringent, diuretic, laxative, digestive, steroid-like.
Indications: throat complaints and bronchitis, renal complaints, constipation, painful periods.
Glycerine macerate of bud ID (Buds*): 30 to 150 drops per day, from the 5th day of the cycle to the next period.

Blackcurrant (*Ribes nigrum*)
Part used: leaves, roots.
Properties: diuretic, eliminator of urea and uric acid, anti-rheumatic, stimulant of the liver, spleen and kidneys, decongestion agent, anti-inflammatory, hormonal regulator: adrenals and ovaries.
Indications: rheumatism, arthritis, migraines, menopause complaints, allergies.

Glycerine macerate of bud ID: 30 to 150 drops per day, except the week of menstrual bleeding.

In *Chinese medicine* there are only two herbs which can be found in our countries:

Ginger
Part used: root.
Ginger is known to us as a digestive, stimulant, tonic or febrifuge. In decoction, fresh ginger is recommended for women having cramps relieved by heat, a white tongue, and a light flow of blackish-red blood during bleeding.

Sage
A herb which imitates the oestrogens and which we will see again shortly in the chapter on irregular periods, page 24. It is recommended for women with abundant, bright red bleeding, abdominal cramps, inclination toward cold and aversion to heat, flushed face, thirst and dehydration, brown and concentrated urine, constipation, and a yellow and furry tongue.

This differentiation comes from the *Barefoot Doctor's Manual* (see References) and is a good example of how to construct the profile of a herb.

To be precise, there are two chemotypes of sage: as an oestrogen-like, salvia sclarea is strong than salvia off.

ॐ 3 ॐ

Irregular Periods

Early periods (8 to 9 days early)

(a) Modern western medicine recognizes three different types of early periods:

(1) Those due to an insufficiency of progesterone. Here ovulation takes place normally; but the second phase is shortened because of an unproductive yellow body (ovary). Treatment: progesterone during the second half of the cycle.

(2) Those due to an early ovulation. In this instance, doctors propose small doses of oestrogen, although the dosage of oestrogen is difficult to calculate, or a few cycles without ovulation (by taking the Pill) in the hopes that the cycle will resume a normal rhythm afterwards.

(3) And those due to an anovular cycle (one without ovulation). This is quite rare, however. Treatment is the administration of Clomid†, to induce ovulation. This drug is known for its occasional triple and quadruple results!

(b) In phytotherapy, there are several oestrogen-like herbs, those which 'imitate' oestrogens.

Sage (*Salvia officinalis*)
Part used: leaves, flowers.
Properties: general tonic, cortico-adrenal stimulant, diuretic,

emmenagogue, digestive, aids conception and childbirth, stops breast milk production, anti-sudoral, hypoglycemiant.

Indications: convalescence, nervous afflictions, asthma, sweats, adenitis, scanty or painful periods, menopause, sterility, preparation for childbirth.

Infusion: 20g (or 2 tablespoons) of leaves and flowers per litre; 3 cups a day.

Tincture: 30 to 40 drops, twice a day.

CAUTION: *essential oil of* salvia officinalis *can bring on epileptic seizures even at low doses. It is therefore preferable to use essential oil*

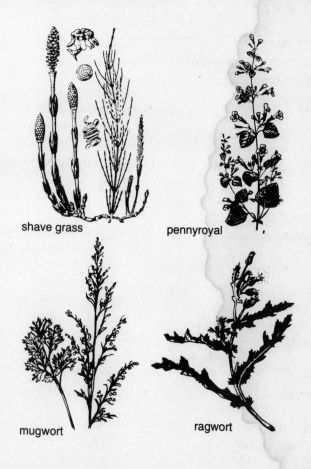

shave grass

pennyroyal

mugwort

ragwort

of salvia sclarea *(which is rich in esters and not in cetones) for internal as well as external use.*

There are also *hormonal regulators* such as blackcurrant and bramble (rubus fructicosus) and sweet briar.

Sweet briar (*rosa canina*)

Part used: flowers, leaves or fruit (rose hips).
Properties: flowers and leaves: laxative, tonic, aids in formation of scars; fruit, additionally: astringent, hemostatic, diuretic, depurative, anti-anaemic.
Indications: leaves and flowers: fatigue, urinary lithiasis, wounds (in external use); fruit: white vaginal discharge, haemorrhage, avitaminosis (lack of vitamins).

It may be noted that *Chinese medicine* also uses sage and sweet briar in the treatment of early periods.

〜

Delayed periods (more than 8 to 9 days overdue)

(a) *Western medicine*

Western medicine attributes oligomenorrhea (cycles of more than 35 days) to three possible causes:

- The excessive persistence of the yellow body, or possibly the formation of an ovarian cyst. *Treatment*: oestrogen, which is intended to inhibit the formation of the yellow body. In the case of a cyst: surgery.
- Late ovulation, which is treated with an agent to induce ovulation, such as clomiphene (Clomid†).
- An anovulary cycle. *Treatment*: inducement of ovulation.

A question we would raise here is whether heavy hormonal treatments don't risk throwing an already disturbed hormonal balance further out of kilter. It seems more prudent, therefore, to avoid their use in endocrinal disturbances such as irregular menstrual periods, and to reserve them for the treatment of major endocrinal syndromes such as Addison's or Cushing's disease.

(b) *Phytotherapy*

In *phytotherapy*, one would use one of the hormonal regulators already discussed:

Raspberry Preferably in glycerine macerate, 50 to 150 drops a day (see also section on disagreeable signs, page 15).
Part used: leaves.
Properties: astringent, diuretic, laxative, digestive.
Indications: rheumatism, arthritis, migraines, menopause complaints, allergies.
Glycerine macerate of bud ID: 50 drops every morning, except the week of menstrual flow.

European ragwort (*Senecio jacobea*)
Part used: entire plant.
Properties: elective action on female genitals, emmenagogue, sedative for menstrual pain, expectorant.
Indications: absence of periods, anaemia, certain types of white vaginal discharge, bronchitis (in external use: tonsillitis, wasp stings, inflammation), throat complaints and bronchitis, renal complaints, constipation, painful periods, irregular cycles.
Decoction: 25g per litre, 2 to 3 cups per day.
Tincture: 20 to 100 drops a day.

In *Chinese Medicine*, sage is used as for early periods, as is angelica, which was discussed in the section on painful periods, page 21. It is clear that these notes offer only a brief glimpse of Chinese medicine since many of the herbs used are not known in the west. It is clear too that the huge domain of acupuncture can only be touched upon here, with a description of the massage of a few pressure points.

Early or delayed periods may pose a problem of sterility or undesired pregnancy for certain women. In particular, irregular or anovular cycles can mean difficulty in conceiving. In regard to this, we would like to present here the work of *Dr Catherine Kousmine*.

Dr Kousmine, of Lausanne, Switzerland, through forty years of research, has demonstrated the connections between nutrition and degenerative diseases (evolutive chronic polyarthritis, multiple sclerosis, and cancer) on the one hand, and the dysfunction of the menstrual cycle and difficulty in conceiving on the other.

Our food is both deficient and too rich. We cannot continue to eat white flour, refined and devoid of all life, and vitamins and minerals, those indispensable catalyzers, or to eat refined sugars (why do you think there is such a demand for dental care in this country?). Food destroyed by our manner of commercialization and preparation cannot be compensated for by 'medical' supplements of calcium, vitamin C, iron, bran . . . in any kind of capsule or pill form.

The functioning of the uterus, the Fallopian tubes, and the ovaries is affected by our diet. For more detailed information, consult the works of Dr Kousmine, paying particular attention to the importance she gives to vitamins E and F.

Vitamin E has an anti-oxydizing function through which it protects polyunsaturated fatty acids (vitamin F), vitamin A, and hypophysial, adrenal and sex hormones, from a premature destruction by oxydation. A lack of vitamin E can increase vitamin and hormonal deficiencies. Vitamin E is scant in foods of animal origin. It is found in green vegetables and especially in nuts and grains, where it is concentrated in the germs and bran. It is eliminated when cereals are sifted, a common practice, but is not destroyed by cooking. The oil of wheat germ is particularly rich in vitamin E.

Vitamin F is the name given to a group of several polyunsaturated fatty acids which regulate the permeability of membranes and are responsible for the synthesis of several elements such as prostaglandins. Linseed, sunflower seed, seeds of *onager* (Oenothera biennis), sesame seed and thistle are particularly rich in vitamin F, but vitamin F survives only in those oils which are entirely cold pressed. Cholesterol, that precious primary substance from which the organism synthesizes vitamin D and sex and adrenal hormones, forms highly soluble salts in the presence of polyunsaturated fatty acids. In their absence, it attaches itself to saturated fatty acids. The salts which result are not readily soluble and precipitate, forming yellow deposits in the skin, mucous membranes or blood veins (an example: a yellow circle visible at the edge of the eye's iris), or in the form of biliary calculus. This is a common phenomenon today among people who consume excessive amounts of animal fats and little raw oil. Among other things, it causes hormonal disturbances.

Coming back to the yoga exercises of Aviva Steiner, mentioned during the discussion on painful periods, there is a sequence specific to ovulation. Certain movements, a certain sequence of exercises, increase the blood flow around the ovary. The ovary is thus better nourished and the Fallopian tubes take on a desirably rhythmic and propulsive tonus. (There is in fact more than one exercise in the 'ovulation' series used to bring on periods, but the 'ovulation' series lasts only 10 minutes, while the first 'menstruation' series lasts 25 minutes, and the second 45!) When the increased blood flow reaches a level where there is congestion, interstitial haemorrhages take place in the uterine mucous membrane which is accustomed to this message at the beginning of each menstrual period. Yes, with these movements, one can bring on periods, even in cases of pregnancy. According to the Israeli women, this method works up until the 10th overdue day.

This brings us to a discussion of delayed periods due to an undesired pregnancy.

We don't intend to stress the method of Aviva here, because it can be difficult to learn when you are already overdue. It takes several months of continuous and somewhat strenuous effort to learn these movements, which means more work than all other existing methods, including Billing's (observation of cervical mucus). The women of the Dutch Women's Health Centres suggest trying to bring on your periods as of the 21st day of the cycle, in order to have several days. It is only when you have been the mistress of these exercises for several months that you can permit yourself to 'dance' only on the day of the expected period, or a little thereafter.

Does it really work? Yes, indeed: the cycle which follows is normal and ovulatory. Heterosexual women do not realize the number of early miscarriages which occur unnoticed (with or without IUD).

But let's return to a more widely known method:

Pennyroyal (*Mentha pulegium*)

Part used: entire plant.

Properties: expectorant, aids evacuation of bile, aids digestion, *emmenagogue*.

Indications: bronchitis, whooping cough, biliary insufficiency, digestive antony (in this, it is like its cousin, mint).

Infusion: 1 teaspoon per cup of water, 3 cups a day for a maximum of 6 days.

CAUTION: *pennyroyal oil is toxic. Symptoms*: nausea and loss of feeling in hands and legs. Two women in Colorado died after ingesting an ounce (33ml) of pennyroyal oil in attempts to self-abort.

Mugwort (*Artemisia vulgaris*)

Part used: entire plant.

Properties: *emmenagogue*, anti-spasmodic, anti-epileptic.

Indications: absence of periods, particularly when connected to anaemia, lymphatism (lymphoid glands increased in volume, softness and thickness), epileptiform accident, nervous complaints, infantile convulsions.

Infusion of leaves or flowers: 1 teaspoon per cup, 3 cups a day, for a maximum of 6 days.

BE CAREFUL NOT TO OVERDOSE: *more than 40g per litre causes hepato-renal disorders and convulsions*.

Contra-indications: uterine inflammation, and recent pelvic infection.

The *Chinese* have known for centuries *the value of mugwort* as a hemostatic and regulator of the menstrual cycle. However it is most commonly used by them to do moxas, that is, to burn a tiny amount of the herb on an acupuncture point.

Black cohosh (*Cimifuga raremosa*)
Part used: root, entire plant.
Properties: reflex moderator of the nervous system, vascular anti-spasmodic, anti-asthmatic, diuretic and *emmenagogue*.
Indications: childbirth, neuralgia, menstrual cramps, muscular cramps aggravated by menstrual periods.
Decoction of the root: boil 1 teaspoon root per cup water. Take three cups a day, for a maximum of 6 days.

Blue cohosh (*Caulophyllum thalictroides*)
Part used: root.
Properties: imitates oxytocin (childbirth hormone), anti-spasmodic, diuretic, *emmenagogue*, sedative.
Indications: aids childbirth, delivery, period pain, childbirth preparation, colic, cramps, rheumatism. Useful in the treatment of spasm as well as uterine atony.
Decoction: 1 teaspoon per cup liquid, 3 cups per day.

In *homoeopathy*, Caulophyllum is used for spasmodic cervical pain in women whose periods are generally light and whose cramps are the worst the first day of menstruation. In 4 or 5 CH, 6 grains every quarter hour, less frequently as soon as there is improvement.

Parsley (*Petroselium sativum*)
Part used: entire plant.
Properties: stimulant, anti-anaemic, depurative, diuretic, regulator of periods, stimulant of smooth muscle fibres (intestines, urinary and biliary canals, uterus).
Indications: anaemia, fatigue, rheumatism, gout, painful periods, cuts breast milk production. In external use: breast engorgement.
Decoction of the entire plant: boil 1 teaspoon per cup liquid for

10 minutes. Take 3 cups per day, or using 50g per litre, 2 to 3 cups per day.

CAUTION: OVERDOSES ARE TOXIC. The seeds are even stronger than the entire plant, and their use is dangerous to, among other things, the kidneys.

Our experience at the Women's Health Center

We have obtained between 60 per cent and 80 per cent effectiveness among women who suspected an undesired pregnancy. Clearly, this figure does not tell us much because we do not know how many of these women were in fact pregnant. The women always used two herbs at a time (most often using either pennyroyal or mugwort, plus one other herb). The best association has been shown to be pennyroyal–blue cohosh.

These herbs seem to be very effective for small delays in menstrual bleeding. Their effectiveness drops noticeably after the 6th day of delay, but still can be useful as long as an inability to confirm the pregnancy makes abortion impossible.

It might be mentioned that these herbs seem *in*effective for periods delayed after going off the Pill, and only slightly effective with irregular cycles.

According to the research and experience of a collective of women in Sante Fe, New Mexico, a better result is obtained with cotton root bark than with pennyroyal. We have therefore integrated this 6th herb into our practice.

Cotton root bark (*Gossypium herbacetum*)
Part used: bark.
Properties: *emmenagogue*, ocytocic.
Indications: childbirth preparation, late periods, painful periods.
Decoction: 1 teaspoon bark per cup liquid for 10 minutes. Take 3 cups per day for a maximum of 6 days.

It is important to note that the earlier the herbs are taken, the more effective they are. There is just one limitation: that the cycle be at its end. Herbs are not effective just after ovulation because it is not possible to loosen mucus which is not yet 'mature'. You can therefore begin to drink infusions the day before the period would normally begin, the same day, or up until the 10th day thereafter. The percentage of success is very good (60–80 per cent) the first 6 days. If you begin drinking the infusions only *after* the 6th day overdue, however, the percentage of effectiveness falls to 20 per cent.

For this reason, after our years of experience, we rarely propose infusions after the 6th day overdue. On the other hand, for those who are among the 20 per cent, it is worth it! The development of early pregnancy tests, however, will probably change our practice and permit a more precise study.

What are the possible side effects? Essentially, contractions whose strength increases in proportion to the length of delay. Sometimes nausea or a light dizziness may result. It is recommended to eat lightly during these days.

Practically speaking
We always prescribe *two* associated herbs (see diagram below).

```
cotton root bark                              parsley
pennyroyal  ──────────── with ──────────  blue cohosh
mugwort                                       black cohosh
```

Using one teaspoonful of each plant, separately, per cup liquid – in infusion for the leaves (mugwort and pennyroyal), and in decoction for the roots (the others) – drink 1 cup of each of the 2 herbs 3 times a day. This means 6 cups to drink each day for a maximum of 6 days.

BE CAREFUL: do not overdose. Do not continue treatment more than six days. Do not begin after the 10th overdue day. The better informed women are, the earlier they will begin. It is not necessary to continue taking the herbs once the period has truly begun.

We might mention a few other emmenagogue herbs: pasque-flower, yarrow, bean trefoil, pineapple, European ragwort, calendula, stachys, germander, southernwood, valerian, rue, aloe, lycopodium, savine, scarlet pimpernel, crocus, ergot of rye, and hyssop.

Self-massage is a good companion treatment to taking herbs. Firstly there is *massage of internal malleolus* on the path of the reflex zones of the uterus along the meridians of the gall bladder-pancreas and liver. This is done following an 'L' in a half-circle around the internal malus as if you were 'following the bed of a river'. Pressure is exerted by the thumb pressing directly *into* the area for 5 minutes on each side, several times a day.

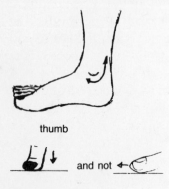

thumb

Secondly, there is another *massage* which is not one a woman can do herself, and which requires a professional masseuse or a trained person with a certain amount of experience. This description will certainly not be sufficient to learn from. It involves deep holds which *tear the connecting tissue* in the areas of stimulation of the reflex zones of the uterus in the lower back, the buttocks, and the upper thigh. If the holds are painful, it means the connecting tissue has been reached, and therefore effective pressure is being exerted.

At the Women's Health Center, we try to do the massage three days in a row at the same time as acupuncture (one and a half hours in all).

A third treatment, therefore, is *acupuncture*. This information will be useful only to those already familiar with acupuncture. **It is not advisable to undertake this treatment unless under expert medical supervision.**

Treatment involves inserting a needle at the 6 gall bladder-pancreas – a point situated on a vertical axis 4 finger widths (fingers of the woman) above the point of the internal malleolus of the two legs – and another at the 4 large intestine on the two hands (with the thumb and index closed, the point is located at the summit of the mound formed by the soft parts).

The needles stay implanted for 30 minutes during which time they are stimulated every 2 minutes by turning them in a clockwise direction until they jam (this may provoke a light local spasm). If during the session the woman succeeds in concentrating on her lower abdomen, she can help the stimulation and feel a sensation of warmth. The contractions can begin during the hour that follows treatment or during the night. Through experience we have realized that these techniques do not work well for women ambivalent about the pregnancy (that is, those who on some level desire it).

As with herbs, the massages and acupuncture are not effective for delays due to an upset of the cycle (the Pill) and amenorrhea.

These last two techniques, massage of connective tissue and acupuncture, are rather difficult and demand a considerable amount of energy from the clinic worker and from the woman involved. According to some clinic workers, these methods may afterwards necessitate the re-establishment of equilibrium, especially where acupuncture was used.

Bleeding

In this section I will discuss both bleeding between periods and over abundant periods. There are so many reasons for bleeding that it is necessary to describe several in order to understand the mechanisms. For this, several questions have to be asked.

Is pregnancy possible? A urine test for pregnancy has

recently been developed which can detect pregnancy as of the 3rd overdue day. (The margin of error is greater from the 3rd to the 12th day.) Some blood tests (available only upon a doctor's prescription) can reveal pregnancy 10 days after conception, that is, before a delay in onset of the menstrual period.

- Find the first day of the last period and count the number of days which have passed. A little bleeding is possible at the moment of the egg's implantation in the lining of the uterus. It is also possible to have a few days' bleeding, a 'false period', which does not interfere with a continued pregnancy.
- Between the 6th and the 10th week, it is possible to have bleeding caused by an insufficiency of the placental shift (the placenta replaces the ovaries in their function of hormonal secretion).
- Another possibility is a spontaneous miscarriage caused by a malformation.
- By the 12th week, most women are aware of being pregnant, and we will not discuss here bleeding which takes place after the first trimester of pregnancy.

For bleeding which takes place during the first three months of pregnancy, even if the pregnancy is desired, few health care workers propose 'preservation' treatment because a high percentage of these pregnancies will not reach full term. (An exception might be the case of repeated miscarriage in a woman desiring a child.)

Whether it is a trace of the blood on the pants, or a false period, bleeding can stop spontaneously. But if the bleeding continues, it is important to note that the *greater the delay, the more difficult it is for the uterus – by itself – to empty itself completely*.

Gynaecologists generally propose a *curettage* to stop bleeding and in order to examine the gathered matter. But if the bleeding is not too abundant, the woman may also treat herself with the help of a utero-contractant such as

Methergin† (ergot of rye, see discussion at the end of this chapter), blue cohosh or essence of lemon. At the risk of protests from specialists, I maintain that a woman who checks herself well can evaluate for herself if the bleeding diminishes normally and whether she has a fever. It is true, however, that if there is any retained matter, she runs the risk of an infection.

Apart from pregnancy, there are numerous causes of bleeding. Let's briefly list the more benign:

- bleeding at *ovulation*. This can be physiological and does not exceed 2–3 days (most often 1–2 days).
- bleeding can come from the bladder; where in doubt, a urine sediment test can be performed. Haemorrhoids should also be considered as a source of bleeding.
- With the aid of a *speculum*, it can be verified whether a lesion of the cervix such as cervicitis is involved.
- Cervical endometriosis (see page 142). The identifying blue patches can be seen more easily at the end of the cycle.
- A *lesion* can be due to a foreign body (forgotten diaphragm, etc.).

If none of these apply, and a severe vaginal infection is not involved (see page 65), the bleeding comes from the uterus.

- Women who have IUDs but do not tolerate them can have intermittent bleeding;
- Women on *the Pill* may have breakthrough bleeding if the oestrogen (first phase) or the progestogen (second phase) do not sufficiently maintain the mucus;
- Otherwise, it may be a matter of *polyps*, growths of placental origin after incomplete childbirth or after an abortion.
- Numerous polyps are a possible consequence of *hyperestrogenemia*. As in the case of a cervical lesion, bleeding can occur after penetration (see Chapter 13 on benign tumours).
- With a *fibroid*, the uterus is enlarged and its muscular fibre no longer has enough elasticity to contract properly (see Chapter 13).

- An *infectious cause* such as endometritis or chronic or acute salpingitis, uterine or tubal tuberculosis, or some other infection (see page 122).
- *Cancer* of the cervic, endocolpitis, or uterus, or, more rarely, of the Fallopian tube or ovary. In this case, bleeding is modest, provoked by contact (sexual intercourse, touch), and can cause anaemia (see page 164).

Be especially alert to bleeding occurring after menopause! How long ago was the last pap smear?

Finally, there are general causes to be considered, such as malnutrition which can cause amenorrhea as well as bleeding, and which is more common than one would think, an endocrinological disorder (thyroid or other), a disease of the blood, or of coagulation, a major metabolic disorder such as diabetes, alcoholism, or cardiac decompensation. To be considered too are *iatrogenic causes*, that is, caused by medicine and medical treatments. An example is the excessive use of hormones, or, to be more specific, Depo-provera. This injectable contraceptive, which lasts for at least three months, has irregular periods and sometimes extremely heavy bleeding as side effects. We might also mention certain neuropsychotropics such as sulpiride (Dogmatil†) and appetite suppressants.

It is evident that a woman cannot answer all these questions herself, and that bleeding may also be a warning of something acute, such as an ectopic pregnancy. It may be prudent therefore to have yourself examined and have a pap smear done (a histological examination of the cervical cells); the situation may even demand a D and C or other surgical intervention.

Where self-treatment is used, therefore, it is important not to go beyond several days of overly abundant bleeding and to evaluate one's condition well.

ॐ

What does modern western medicine propose?

This will be brief because there is enough information elsewhere on this subject.

Depending on the state of the endometrium, the abundance of the bleeding, and the drugs available:

- compensation for the loss of blood;
- curettage, as much a treatment as an aid to diagnosis;
- oestrogen;
- a progesteron, if the cycle is anovulatory;
- androgens (testosterone) for those women over 45 years of age (although women of this age are already producing less oestrogen than earlier in their lives with a resulting shift to proportionally more androgens);

Longer-term measures:

- clomiphene (Clomid†);
- androgens again;
- thyroid hormones, if they are low;
- chorionic gonadotrophins (HCG), if it is the second phase which is shortened before the bleeding;
- prednisone, in certain cases of reduced bleeding (Stein-Leventhal syndrome);
- surgery (hysterectomy: removal of the uterus), when they don't know what else to do.

This list is hardly tempting, I fully agree, so let's return to the *alternatives*, especially those concerned with *over-abundant periods*:

Since menstrual periods are an opportunity for the organism to eliminate toxins, you can begin by asking yourself just what you ate during the cycle preceding menstrual bleeding. Too much meat? Any binges? The number of consultations for abdominal pain, painful periods, bleeding . . . after 'celebrations' is something all health care workers are familiar with!

⌇

The herbs

Blue cohosh See page 31.

Shave grass (*Equisetum arvense*)
Part used: stem or entire plant.
Widely recognized for its remineralizing properties, shave grass is also a diuretic, a hemostatic and aids in the formation of scar tissue.
Indications: Among its numerous indications are: cystitis, albuminermia, haemorrhage, including breakthrough bleeding, demineralization (tuberculosis, rickets, fractures).
Powder: 1 teaspoon in a little water before or after the two main meals (may be taken in capsule or tablet form).
Tincture: 20 to 50 drops, twice a day.

⌇

The essential oils

Lemon
Part used: fruit, essential oil (EO).
Among the numerous properties of lemon: bactericide and antiseptic, alcalinizing gastric antacid, anti-arthritis, lowers hyperviscosity of the blood, depurative, aids hepatic, pancreatic and gastric secretions, hemostatic.
Indications: infection, hypergastric acidity, difficult digestion, hepatic insufficiency and congestion, haemorrhage.
In this last indication (bleeding), EO: 10–15 drops 3 times per day after meals in a solution of alcohol-glycerine or in a hysolisant of soya (see proportions in Appendix 2, page 211).

For other indications: lemon juice cure, ½ to 10 lemons per day, progressively increasing the quantity (½ the first day, 1 the second, etc.) until you reach the maximum number of lemons, after which you begin decreasing the quantity.

Cinnamon (*Cinnamomum z.*)
Part used: bark and EO of bark and leaves.
Properties: stimulant, antiseptic, anti-spasmodic, hemostatic, (aphrodisiac), emmenagogue.
Indications: weakness, aches or fever, flu, digestive spasms, breakthrough bleeding, scanty periods.
EO: 2–3 drops, twice a day in an alcohol-glycerine solution.

Cypress (*Cupressus*)
Part used: entire plant.
Properties: astringent, vaso-constrictor, anti-spasmodic, anti-sudorific, anti-rheumatic, diuretic.
Indications: haemorrhoids, varicose veins, painful periods, bleeding, menopause.
Tincture: 30 to 60 drops before the two main meals.
EO: 2–4 drops, 2–3 times a day in an alcohol-glycerine solution.

Geranium (*Pelargonium odorantissimum*)
Part used: entire plant.
Properties: tonic, astringent, hemostatic, antiseptic.
  In external use: aids scar formation, antalgic, mosquito repellent, anti-coagulant.
Indications: fatigue, gastroenteritis, uterine haemorrhage, sterility, urinary lithiasis, gastric ulcer.
Infusion: 1 teaspoon per cup liquid, 3 cups a day.
EO: 2–4 drops, 2–3 times a day.

But no chapter on the herbs indicated in case of bleeding would be complete without the story of *ergot of rye*, a parasite of rye.

Ergot has been recognized and used for centuries as the key utero-contractant for all bleeding. It was used so often that finally there were too many accidents: ruptured uteri caused by a disproportion of the diameter of the head/pelvis during childbirth, and poisonings. The School of Medicine in Geneva has, since 1800, recommended its use only when the uterus is empty – that is, outside of labour, delivery and abortion! Ergot certainly has an action on the smooth muscle fibres such as the uterus, arteries, bladder, bronchial tubes and the stomach. But when overdosed and poorly indicated, the uterus contracts while the cervix closes and thus retention takes place. Ergot of rye is used as an allopathic remedy, available only on prescription, in the form of Methergin†. After having been widely used, its administration in the follow-up of abortion and childbirth is presently under criticism.

৵

Chinese medicine uses other herbs

Peony (*Paeonia off.*)
Active part: flowers and roots.

An ancient remedy for epilepsy, peony is an anti-spasmodic and indicated in hyperexcitability (an anxious type of person who is bothered by palpitations).

Tincture: 30–50 drops per day.

(*Poterium sanguisorba*)
Part used: entire plant.

Poterium sanguisorba has been known since ancient times as an astringent in hematurias (blood in the urine), spitting of blood, breakthrough bleeding, haemorrhoids, and diarrhoea. It is little known to today's herbalists; it is mentioned by one author for relief of severe diarrhoea (Leclerc).

Thuja (*Thuja occidentalis*) or 'tree of life'
Part used: leaves, bark.

Properties: light diuretic and urinary sedative, expectorant, sudorific, anti-rheumatism, anti-cancer.

Indications: cystitis, pelvic congestion, rheumatism, cancerous state.

In external use: warts, condylomas and polyps.

Orally: tincture of ⅕: 20–40 drops per day.

External use: EO or tincture applications twice a day.

In homoeopathy, thuja is an important remedy of cycosis (result of gonorrhea). It is a ground remedy. At the genital level, it is indicated in inflammatory states: warts, condylomas, polyps, irritating white, evil-smelling and greenish-white secretions, infection of the uterus and adjoining areas, especially on the left side, and pain at penetration and during periods. Thuja is also a remedy for fibroids and cysts, and is used in the treatment of cancer.

For local use: 7 to 9 CH, 1 dose 3 times per week. Generally, however, thuja is used as a ground remedy, and dosed at a higher dilution (see homoeopathy literature).

Clove (*Eugenia caryophyllata*)

Part used: bud of the flower ('cloves'), or essential oil of clove.

Properties: excitant, uterine tonic, antiseptic, aids digestions, anti-neuralgic, anti-spasmodic, anti-cancer. In the west, clove is not recognized as indicated in uterine bleeding, although sucking on a clove is used in childbirth preparation (!), prevention of infectious diseases, difficult digestion, and dental neuralgia.

EO: 2–4 drops, 3 times a day.

In childbirth preparation: use clove as a flavouring in food in the final months of pregnancy. At the approach of each term: infusion of clove, using an additional clove with each passing day.

The *Chinese* use black cohosh (see Chapter 2 on painful periods), and mugwort, which we know as an emmenagogue. For still other herbs, see section on bleeding in cases of fibroids, pages 155–6.

4

Menopause

Once we understand what kinds of changes take place in the menopause, we should be able to approach it without fear. That is the first goal of this chapter, since talking about menopause is still taboo!

A woman's cultural context is an important factor in how she experiences menopause. In our western countries, where youth and motherhood are overemphasized in comparison to a woman's professional, artistic or other abilities, and where women are primarily considered sex objects, women too often regard menopause as the end of their lives. Other events coincide with this end of having children, such as the death of a husband or a lover, a greater difficulty in finding paid employment, or perhaps the loss of paid employment, contributing to the stress of this period of change.

However, menopause marks only the end of fertility, it is not the end of life or all productivity, nor is it the end of sexuality.

When a woman is unable to share her experiences or learn about other women's experiences, she may easily blame herself for any difficulties which may arise. Along with sexuality (and money!) menopause is one of the first subjects around which women need an exchange of experiences, information, and support (a self-help group).

According to an American source (*Health Right*, New York, 1976), 10 per cent of all women experience no disagreeable signs at the approach of menopause; 80 per cent do, but find

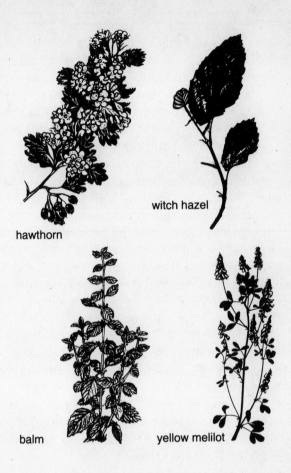

hawthorn

witch hazel

balm

yellow melilot

them tolerable; and the remaining 10 per cent find the signs too disagreeable and ask for medication.

Disagreeable signs associated with menopause

Before menopause, that is, the definitive disappearance of menstrual periods, there is a period of great hormonal changes in the body which may last several years. The ovaries secrete fewer and fewer oestrogens and progesterone. During this period of progressively decreased production, there are moments of marked imbalance between these two hormones. The production of oestrogens does not stop completely; small quantities continue to be secreted by the adrenals until about the age of 70. The body has to adapt to these changes and does so in a fashion which is at times chaotic.

Some of the disagreeable signs, and there is a great variety, are provoked by the brusque imbalance between the hormones. But there are also those which are linked to a general state of health: weaknesses, amount of reserve strength, and a wearing out of the body, as well as self-image, social role and personal expectations.

(Incidentally, it is recommended to wait at least a year after the definitive end of periods before ceasing to use contraceptives!)

Let's take a look at these signs:

- menstrual irregularity: shortening of the cycle and diminution of menstrual flow, or lengthening of the cycle and increased flow;
- hot flushes, at first at night, provoked by the warmth of the bed, and possibly accompanied by leg cramps. Hot flushes also occur during the course of the day as well, especially after a meal or physical effort. Hot flushes occur most often before the periods and are stronger if the periods are delayed;
- congestion of the lower abdomen: bloating, difficult digestion, migraine, constipation, urinary infections, increased vaginal secretions, haemorrhoids;
- sudden change of character: aggression, mood swings, insomnia or anxiety, depression, compulsive eating;
- circulatory troubles: most frequent are vascular problems: heavy legs, cramps, varicose veins; more rarely: hypertension, angina;
- bone disorders, depending on the state of the bones and cartilages and on the body's capacity to retain calcium: disks

pinched between the vertebrae, stiffening in joints, fallen arches;
* sore breasts with hypersensitive masses;
* easily broken nails, dry skin, fragile mucous membranes (for example, the vagina and vulva).

Rest assured, you will never have all of them at the same time!

&

What does modern western medicine propose?

* information;
* sedatives, tranquillizers, sleeping pills.

Specifically:

* hormone replacement therapy, aiming for an effective minimal dose, e.g. Premarin† (conjugated oestrogens of equine origin), 0.3, 0.625, or 1.25mg per day, 20 days out of 30.
  Other possibilities: diethylstilbestrol (DES!!! see page 49) or ethinyloestradiol or finally a more recent form, the patch (skin adhesive), Oestraderm TTS†, eventually associated to progesteron the few days before the periods;
* androgens, such as methyltestosterone (watch out for masculinization!);
* other oestrogens and androgens.

For confirmed menopause: same as above, plus oestrogens and progesterone (such as the Pill).
CAUTION: *breast and pelvic examinations for tumours are vital!!*
   Local treatment (vulvar or vagina): DES in ovules or in cream form, androgen in tabs or Premarin† cream.

Treatment for osteoporosis:

- calmative, codeine, aspirin;
- hormonal therapy;
- diet: increase protein intake and vitamin D.

༄

The controversy over replacement hormones

Since the advertising department of the pharmaceutical multinationals have succeeded so well in creating a 'need' for hormone replacement during menopause, it is important to devote some time here to their advantages and disadvantages.

In presenting the precursor signs of menopause as 'symptoms', or as a 'syndrome', the pharmaceutical multinationals would have us believe that menopause is an illness. Now they have only to convince large numbers of women that replacement oestrogens can prevent osteoporosis and cardio-vascular illness while guaranteeing 'eternal youth'!

Of course, to do this, they will need to avoid mentioning the *risks* that taking hormones presents (for example, the risk of cancer of the uterus goes from 5 per cent to 15 per cent for a woman who has taken oestrogens for more than five years[1]), or the possible *side effects*: nausea, thromboses, phlebitis, gall bladder disease, headaches, and depression.

It is a little hard to believe that oestrogens prevent cardio-vascular diseases when it is known that – on the contrary – it aggravates them: oestrogens during pregnancy aggravate varicose veins and the Pill is contra-indicated in hypertension! In addition, osteoporosis is not an inevitable consequence of ageing (see box, page 50). The women of the National Women's

---

[1] These results are from studies involving the prescription of often high dosages of oestrogen alone. Risks are far less if oestrogen is given with a progestogen.

Health Network (USA), allied with feminist groups and consumer groups, won a trial in 1977 which compelled the manufacturers of oestrogens to include a notice in each package enumerating the product's risks and possible side effects, as well as its positive effects. Osteoporosis is not included among the possibilities listed on this notice, only the 'tonic' effect on the breasts and on hair growth!

But since the end of the 1980's, with the discovery of 'patches' and creams for the cutaneous absorption of hormones (Oestroderm TTS), we have seen a new offensive for hormone replacement by the multinational pharmaceutical corporations. We are told once again that oestrogen lowers the risk of cardio-vascular disease and is an excellent preventative against osteoporosis! Side effects are minimized because this time we are supposed to take oestrogen as soon as we reach 40 and thereafter until the end of our lives!!

But our question remains. Does oestrogen cause cancer? . . .

Do oestrogens cause cancer? This question has already caused a lot of ink to be spilt. We ourselves are certain of but one thing – that existing cancer can be aggravated by oestrogens. Doctors, at least, have been warned about this, but have the women for whom replacement hormones are being prescribed?

A few words on DES (diethylstilbestrol), which has been implicated in cancer and anomalies of the vagina and cervix, as well as a higher rate of miscarriage in some daughters of women treated with it at the beginning of their pregnancy. In Switzerland, DES was commercially available under the name of Hormoestrol†. In the US, DES was largely used as the 'morning-after' pill, with a large number of failures and side effects. When we see how DES and the Pill have been introduced on the market, by removing from studies those laboratory animals with tumours in order to hide this risk and to see the incidence of tumours reappear in thousands of women at their expense, we can be forgiven a certain mistrust today. In the UK, fortunately, DES was little used as a treatment, during pregnancy or as a 'morning-after' pill.

ॐ

Oestrogens and osteoporosis

During the first months of oestrogen treatment, a drop in urinary elimination of calcium can be noticed in menopausal and osteoporotic women. However, while oestrogens diminish bone destruction, bone tissue renewal does not increase (and may even decrease). Oestrogens produce a retention of calcium and delay somewhat the progression of osteoporosis, but they cannot restore the bone mass. In addition, the effectiveness of the treatment decreases over time.

Generally, good bone growth depends on:

- the presence of minerals in sufficient quantity (calcium, phosphorus . . .);
- vitamin D (therefore, its absorption by the digestive tube and through the sun on the skin, and its activation by the kidneys);
- a balance between bone formation and destruction, which is determined especially by the parathyroid hormones and by calcitonin;
- other hormones which ossify: androgens and thyroid hormones (those which destroy the bone and inhibit its growth are the corticoid hormones);
- a healthy circulatory system which in turn is linked to physical exercise.

Today thanks to mineralmetry, we can measure precisely the bone density of the femur and the base of the spine. Bone density is measured in percentages according to age group. In our practice, we have shown that it is possible to remineralize a woman, after menopause and without hormone replacement therapy, through dietary changes, remineralizing agents, and, of course, changes in lifestyle.

Note: consumption of sugar uses the calcium upon which bones depend.

Another general disadvantage of replacement hormones is that the weaning from them often leads to a renewal of disagreeable signs similar to those replacement hormones were meant to suppress. So unless you plan to take them your entire life, you merely defer the signs. Important, too, is that the risks of hormonal replacement increase with prolonged use (more than five years). It is true, however, that many women have found relief by taking hormones, often not having had a choice. We are among those who think that if one chooses to take oestrogens, then it is best to associate them with a progestogen in the second phase of the (simulated) cycle, as this diminishes the risks, but if you add progesteron, you have periods and more side effects (particularly in the digestive and circulatory system)! In our experience, replacement hormones are often difficult to dose; for this reason, we prefer to leave this task to the specialists.

In conclusion, let's go over the *contra-indications* for replacement hormones: blood which has a tendency to clot, thrombosis, hypertension, heart, liver and kidney diseases, diabetes, tuberculosis, anaemia, cancer, benign tumours such as fibroids and cysts in breasts.

ॐ

There is, however, another approach

For certain women, the best treatment for the disagreeable signs of menopause is to stay active, to feel useful, to love and to be loved. Being above all a matter of 'well-being', continued physical exercise, sexual expression, and orgasms certainly play an important role. Indeed, one of the things which doctors never tell women is that the best way to combat the shrinking and drying of the vagina is to continue to have orgasms!

Nutrition is also of great importance. A diet is needed which is rich in proteins (note: vegetable proteins are more digestible than animal proteins), and minerals and vitamins (especially vitamin D), which are found in whole grains, in raw fruits and vegetables, and in cold pressed oils eaten uncooked on food (sunflower, wheat germ, thistle or linseed cut with another oil). We will come back to diet and to the food preparation which best preserves the richness of food in Chapter 15.

ॐ

At the risk of repeating ourselves, a diet rich in what?

In vitamins

Vitamin E: vitamin of the genital sphere *par excellence*, but also of the cardio-vascular and neuro-muscular systems and of the skin, vitamin E is particularly indicated in vulvatisis, vulvar itching and genital disorders of menopause. It is found in grains, especially in their germs, and in cold pressed oils, the green part of vegetables, pollen and peanuts.

Vitamin F: Essential fatty acids little known and none the less of capital importance, this name regroups three non-saturated acids which are present in all the cells and which intervene in the synthesis of fats. Its role is essential in cellular exchange; it is, in fact, an excellent anti-toxic vitamin. A deficiency of vitamin F causes dermatoses, circulatory, liver and nervous problems, and predisposes one to cancer. It is found in virgin cold pressed oils: sunflower, walnut, hazelnut, colza, thistle and linseed (the last of these having the strongest taste);

Vitamin A: a growth vitamin involved in the production of cells of the skin, mucous membranes and scar tissue, it is found in fish, milk products, lettuce, spinach, carrots, and apricots.

Vitamin B: a complex including some 20 vitamins essential for growth, nerves, eyes, skin and mucous membranes. B1 and B3 are useful in cases of headaches, B2 in vaginal itching, B6 in cramps, and B9 or folic acid in the formation of oestrogens. They are found in brewer's yeast, wheat germ, and, in general, in whole grains, almonds, fish, salmon, meat and liver.

And in minerals

Calcium: acts against osteoporosis and hot flushes, in conjunction with vitamin C. It is found in milk products, mustard, dandelion, watercress, almonds and sesame seeds.

Iron: this indispensable constituent of haemoglobin which intervenes in the oxygenation of tissues and in anaemia is found in molasses, parsley, spinach, eggs, apricots, red beets and whole grains. Iron is absorbed only in the presence of copper, which is found in fresh fruits and green vegetables. In trace elements, the association is Mn-Cu-Co (manganese, copper, cobalt). One of the easiest ways to rapidly increase your intake of iron is to eat each day an apple into which several nails of oxydizable iron have been put the night before (a recipe borrowed from our prenatal care experience). Take the nails out before biting it!

Magnesium (Mg) has an enzymatic function and is necessary to the absorption of calcium. It is a cellular regenerator, psychological and vaso-sympathic system (the source of hot flushes) equilibrator, and a hepatic drainer. Mg fights ageing. It is found in: soya, nuts, whole grains, sea salt, milk, eggs and lemon.

Phosphorus: plays a role in the formation of tissue between bones, in the production of hormones, and in the absorption of calcium. It is a prime element of nervous, intellectual and sexual energy. It is found in: grains, wheat germ, garlic, celery, carrots, sesame, almonds, walnuts, grapes and fish.

On the herbal side

- For hot flushes:
  In glycerine macerate of bud ID (ID: the first tenth of a
  10 per cent solution): mistletoe and blackcurrant;
  In tincture: blackcurrant, rose hips, water lily, sage,
  climbing ivy, balm and witch hazel.
- *In essential oil*: basil, thyme and hops.
- For low abdominal congestion: drainers, of course, and

digestive regulators. *Tincture*: artichoke, boldo, condurango, combretum, rosemary, turmeric, dandelion, and shave grass.

- For circulatory disorders: *tincture*: hazelnut, cowped, meadowsweet, yellow melilot, bilberry, blackcurrant and witch hazel.
- For nervousness and sleep disorders: *in infusion or tincture*: yellow melilot, sweet clover, passion flower, linden tree flower, willow, peony, balm, hawthorn and hops.
- For problems concerning elasticity of the vagina: *in local use*: vitamin E, essential oil of *salvia sclarea* and cypress, lactate of Mg, seaweed and clay in the form of a vaginal suppository (see page 118).

What to do with all this? Certain naturopaths propose a preparation of 15 herbs, including almost all of these we have just seen. Others think that, even if their actions complete and amplify one another, it is preferable to use no more than 4 to 5 herbs per preparation. Finally, to know the precise action of a plant it is preferable to try one at the time.

So, how do you choose them? By reading a profile of each herb in a book on phytotherapy, and seeing which ones 'resemble' you the most in their other properties and indications.

But let's look at these herbs more closely
Hops (*Humulus lupulus*)
Part used: female flowers, fruits, cones.
Properties: oestrogen-like, tonic, aperitif, digestive, genital sedative, hypnotic, diuretic and depurative.
Indications: convalescence, anaemia, stomach pain, white discharge, cervical inflammation, dermatose and insomnia.
Infusion: 30g of cones for 1 litre, 3 cups a day
Tincture: 20 to 80 drops per day.

Yellow melilot (*Melitotus off.*)
Part used: flower tops.
Properties: anti-spasmodic, calmative of the sympathetic nervous system, sedative, urinary antiseptic, anti-coagulant.

Indications: insomnia, nervousness, depression, spasmodic coughs, urinary ailments, disorders of menopause, phlebitis. In external use: eye ailments.
Infusion: 1 teaspoon per cup liquid, 2 to 3 cups a day.
Tincture: 45 to 90 drops a day.

In homoeopathy, *melitotus* is indicated in acute local congestion, principally in the head, with flushed face and throbbing headache.

Witch hazel (*Hamamelis virginiana*)
Part used: leaves, bark of young stems.
Properties: vaso-constrictor, improves elasticity of veins, circulatory regulator, analgesic, haemostatis, astringent.
Indications: affected veins (varicose veins, haemorrhoids, phlebitis, leg ulcers), uterine, ovarian, and pelvic congestion, haemorrhage, menopause, itching.
Decoction: boil 1 teaspoon of herb in 1 cup liquid for ten minutes. Drink 2 cups per day.
Tincture of ⅕: 20 drops, 3 times a day.

In homoeopathy, *hamamelis* is known for its action on the vein system and is used for varicose veins, haemorrhoids, and haemorrhage (with black blood), especially post-trauma.

Sage (*Salvia off.*) See page 24, section on irregular periods.

Cypress (*Cupressus*)
Part used: cones, leaves, fruit.
Properties: vaso-constrictor and vein tonic, anti-spasmodic, decreases perspiration, re-balances nervous system.
Indications: haemorrhoids, varicose veins, ovarian disorders, menopause, rheumatism.

Ginseng (that centuries-old Chinese panacea)
Part used: root.
Properties: stimulant, revitalizer, vaso-motor, digestive, antalgic in rheumatism.
Indications: physical and intellectual fatigue, convalescence, lack

of appetite, ageing, vascular ailments, psychosomatic illnesses.
Decoction of root: 0.5g per dose.
Tincture: 20 drops, 3 times a day for 4 to 6 weeks.

Currently very fashionable, the quality of that which can be bought in the west is unfortunately not always up to standard. In the west, some herb sellers say that there are western herbs which are just as powerful, such as rosemary, and that it is in any case preferable to use a local herb.

Balm (*Melissa off.*)
Part used: flower tops and leaves.
Properties: tonic action on the brain, heart, uterus, digestive organs; anti-spasmodic, physical and intellectual stimulant; aids periods.
Indications: migraines, neuralgia, nervous breakdown, spasm (asthma), loss of memory, depression, indigestion, painful periods.
Infusion: 1 teaspoon per cup liquid, 3 cups per day.
Tincture: 40 drops after meals.

Hawthorn (*Crataegus oxycantha*)
Part used: flowers and buds.
Properties: cardiac tonic, hypotensor through vasodilation, anti-spasmodic, astringent.
Indications: palpitations, heart pain, angina, vascular spasm, congestive flushes, menopausal insomnia, neuro-vegetative dystony (anxiety, dizziness, ringing in the ears).
Infusion: 1 teaspoon per cup liquid, 2 to 3 cups a day.
Tincture: 20 to 60 drops a day.

Trace-elements

Here is the opportunity to introduce a therapeutic agent which we haven't yet mentioned.

Trace-elements are metals suspended in a liquid solution. Present in the organism in trace form, they aid certain enzymatic reactions.

Studies have demonstrated the connection between trace-elements and certain metabolic disorders (see References and Appendix 3 on the diatheses in the use of trace-elements).

The trace-elements which interest us here are:

- copper-gold-silver (Cu-Au-Ag), the association of trace-elements of infectious states, lethargic fatigue, and convalescence;
- zinc-copper (Zn-Cu) or zinc-nickel-cobalt (Zn-Ni-Co), the association of trace-elements in functional endocrinological disorders;
- magnesium (Mg), which we saw earlier in this chapter, when diet was discussed.

Trace-elements are taken in the morning before breakfast. Two to three times a week, place the liquid under your tongue. Let it warm in your mouth 2 minutes, then swallow. After several weeks, they no longer have an effect. Spacing out treatments and stopping from time to time permits a renewal of beneficial action.

ॐ 5 ॐ

Amenorrhea

The true cause of an absence of menstrual periods, amenorrhea, is difficult to pinpoint because of the number of factors which come into play in the regulation of periods.

The hypothalamus (a little understood cerebral gland) influences the pituitary gland, also known as the hypophysis. The pituitary gland, situated in the middle of the brain, influences the ovary through the hormones which it secretes (FSH, LH). The ovary, through its secretion of oestrogens and progesterons, influences the uterus and breasts . . . and the increased concentration of these hormones in the blood influences in turn the hypothalamus and the pituitary gland (see page 10).

In the same way, the adrenals, the thyroid and the pancreas influence the pituitary gland, which in turn influences them. Thus, in the hormonal inter-play there is always a mechanism of circular feedback. This feedback information acts as a brake on the secretion of hormones, keeping each in balance in relation to the others. The equilibrium thus created depends equally on each side of the links of the hormonal chain.

In medicine a distinction is made between primary and secondary amenorrhea.

Primary amenorrhea: periods which have never been established. This is rare, but can be found in cases of certain malformations of the adrenals, the caryotype (or chromosomal code),

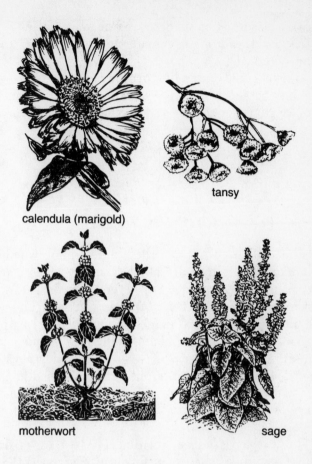

calendula (marigold)

tansy

motherwort

sage

vaginal anatomy such as atresia, or strangling of the cervix, scar tissue as a result of tuberculosis or an accident, or in a delayed development of the pituitary gland or ovary.

Secondary amenorrhea: the disappearance of periods. This condition can be traced to:

- general causes: tuberculosis, cyrrhosis, thyroid insufficiency, adrenal diseases, and dietary deficiency;
- uterine causes: the same as those in primary amenorrhea, and trauma or post-infection scar tissue;
- iatrogenic causes (caused by the intervention of medical practices): in particular, after going off the Pill!

- ovarian causes: tumour or cyst of the ovary (Stein-Leventhal syndrome), premature menopause; and, the most frequent,
- pituitary gland causes: life changes such as travel, emotional shock, or loss or gain of a considerable amount of weight (more than 10 or 15 pounds).

ᘓ

What does modern western medicine propose?

First, a diagnostic test in order to determine whether the failure to bleed is 'true' amenorrhea: an intra-muscular injection of progesterone, once or several days in a row (for a maximum of 5 days). Then, if that doesn't work, an injection of DES (! see page 49) (though not in the UK), 1mg per day for 3 weeks. Until the beginning of the 1980s, Duogynon† or Cumorit† (an association of oestrogens and progestogens: ethinyloestradial/noresthisterone) was prescribed in Europe. These, like DES, are contraindicated during pregnancy, and after years of controversy were finally withdrawn from the market.

The next step is induce ovulation. The best-known drug for this is Clomid†, 50mg per day for 5 days. Pergonal† (FSH and LH) can also be used in intra-muscular injections for 6 to 12 days, followed by HCG, also by injection, until ovulation.

In addition, there are of course rare problems which require surgery or the treatment of a general cause (see above).

ᘓ

And natural healing?

The importance of *diet* cannot be stressed enough. In questioning women who complain of even short spells of amenorrhea, their diet turns out to be clearly marked by nutritional deficiencies – despite the women's assertions that they eat 'normally'. See Chapter 3 on irregular periods, as well as Chapter 15 on diet.

In the experience of Dr Catherine Kousmine, who has treated a number of these women, it takes two years to re-establish a cycle through diet until, for example, conception is possible. She has also documented the frequency of deficiencies in iron in these women. See the section on menopause, page 53.

჻

But let's turn to the herbs

The regularizers of the pituitary gland
- The oestrogen-like plants and those which stimulate the cortico-adrenals*. *Essential oils*: savory, parsley, thyme, borneol, geranium, hops, nutmeg, basil, oregano, cypress, camomile and mint. *Tincture*: calendula, sage, European ragwort, currant, liquorice, cones of hops, climbing ivy, raspberry, thorn, mugwort and arnica.
- The progesterone-like plants (those which imitate progesterone): gromwell, stoneseed, meadowsweet, tansy, yarrow, sarsaparilla, chaste tree and lady's mantel.

EO *salvia sclarea*	3g
EO *salvia off.*	2g
EO *cypres semp.*	8g
EO *mugwort arb.*	2g
EO *lavender off.*	8g

Massage the ovarian area until absorption, eventually mixed with almond oil.
- To rebalance the ground and drain the eliminatory organs (kidneys, intestines, liver, lungs, skin), the 'purges' of traditional medicine: shave grace (especially good), rose hips, lemon, rosemary, artichoke, boldo, fumitory,

condurango, honey and pollen. *Trace elements*: cobalt, copper, zinc, manganese, lithium and magnesium.

- To facilitate local and general circulation, if it is a weak point in the woman: witch hazel, goldenseal, hazel tree, cowped, ruscus, periwinkle, yellow melilot and scarlet pimpernel.
- To calm the central nervous system and the neuro-vegetative system, if there is need: *essential oil*: neroli, angelica, tarragon, lavender. *Tincture*: sweet clover, willow, black horehound, hawthorn, anemone, passion flower, valerian, peony, gelsemium, and balm.

Once again, a long list of herbs. What are you supposed to do with all that? You can begin quite simply by taking a *tincture of sage*, 50 drops twice a day. When you begin to bleed, decrease the *tincture of sage* to 30 drops in the morning, and add 50 drops of glycerine macerate of raspberry bud in the evenings, in order to regularize the cycle and avoid painful periods.

To be a little more sophisticated, you can try to 'construct a cycle' by taking oestrogen-like herbs with a drainer or other ground herb during the first phase; and the in second phase, progesterone-like herbs with circulatory and tranquillizer herbs, for example.

We have already looked at sage on page 24 and shave grass on page 40. Let's take a look at a few new herbs now.

Calendula or Marigold (*Calendula off.*)
Part used: flowers.

Properties: regulator of periods and calmative of their pain, depurative, diuretic, hypotensor, stimulant, antiseptic, aids in the formation of scar tissue (an excellent remedy for wounds).

Indications: scanty menstrual flow, painful periods, hepatic congestion, gastric and intestinal ulcers, cancer (uterus, stomach). *In external use*: wounds, ulcers and abscesses.

Tincture: 60 to 120 drops a day.

In external use: decoction or tincture: dilute 1 teaspoon in a bowl of water.

Tansy (*Tanacetum vulgare*)
Part used: entire plant, flower tops.
Properties: vermifuge, anti-spasmodic, aids in menstrual flow, tonic, febrifuge, antiseptic, progesterone-like.
Indications: oxyures, ascaris, spasmodic colitis, scanty menstrual flow, weakness, fever state.
Infusion of seeds and flowers: 1 teaspoon per cup liquid, 3 cups a day.
Water extract: 0.2 to 0.6g per day, only in the second phase.

Stoneseed (*Lithospermum ruderdale*)
Here in Europe we know only *lithospermum off.* (gromwell) which is a diuretic and dissolvant of calculus. But native North Americans have long used lithospernum ruderdale as a contraceptive herb! A maceration of the root, taken over a long period of time, seems to function, progesterone-like, as an inhibitor of the pituitary gland. For use in cases of amenorrhea, dilute a tincture to 10 per cent in a tincture of alcoholate of olive (the plant). Take 30–50 drops per day, more in the second phase than in the first.

Lavender (*Lavanda vera*)
Part used: flower.
Properties: anti-spasmodic, analgesic, antiseptic and bactericide, aids in secretion of bile, diuretic, tonic, emmenagogue.
Indications: infectious illnesses, particularly those of the respiratory passages, irritability, depression, migraines, cystitis, scanty menstrual flow. *In external use*: vaginal discharge, fungus, wounds, burns, insect bites.
Infusion: 1 teaspoon per cup liquid, 3 cups a day.
Essential oil: 2 to 4 drops, 3 times a day in an alcohol/glycerine solution or in soya (see Appendix 2).

Rosemary (*Rosmarinus off.*)
Properties: general stimulant (tonicardiac, stimulant of cordico-adrenals), hypertensor, pulmonary antiseptic, aids in secretion of bile, emmenagogue.
Indications: fatigue, asthma, migraine, difficult digestion, painful periods and vaginal discharge.

Infusions: as usual.
Tincture: 30–120 drops a day.
Essential oil: 3 to 4 drops per day in an alcohol solution or in
   honey, after meals.

CAUTION: at high doses essential oil of rosemary triggers
epileptic seizures and can provoke haemorrhages, albumin-
imia, and a fatty degeneration of the liver and kidneys.

Certain herbs used in Chinese medicine are known to us:
thuja, mentioned on page 42, selaginelle, of which there are
600 different species in Europe, including one which grows in
the Swiss Alps (!), although western medicine does not recognize it as a medicinal herb, and rhubarb, which is not known to
us as having a gynaecological use. It is used in anaemia, general
weaknesses, and digestive problems. It is contra-indicated in
haemorrhoids, gout and renal illnesses (oxalic lithiasis).

Motherwort (*Leonorus cardiaca*)
Part used: flower tops and leaves.
Properties: anti-spasmodic, emmenagogue, calmative for the
   nerves, laxative.
Indications: palpitations, angina, amenorrhea, urinary cramp,
   albumin in the urine, congestive states, painful periods and
   anaemia.
Decoction: 3 cups a day.

If these treatments don't work, you should try a ground
treatment in energetic acupuncture (see page 34) or in
homoeopathy. Homoeopathy is particularly useful if periods
stop after an emotional trauma (e.g. grief, miscarriage,
breaking up).

๖ 6 ๖

Vaginal and Vulvar Infections

๖

The vagina is normally the home of a wide range of bacteria. The most numerous of these are the lactic bacteria whose presence renders the milieu acid. It is this acidity which protects the vagina from all kinds of pathological germs. If, for one reason or another (see below), the ecological balance of the vagina is disturbed, fungus, protozoa (one-celled organisms) and bacteria can overgrow, causing discharges of varying colour, consistency and odour, as well as a burning sensation and painful itching.

๖

What can change the ecological balance of the vagina?

Our vagina is not an isolated organ which the gynaecologist examines. It is a part of our body and whatever happens to us (physically and emotionally) can have an effect on our health. We are more likely to catch an infection if our resistance has been weakened by:

- another infection
- an unbalanced diet
- a lack of sleep

- anaemia
- drugs (for example, antibiotics)
- certain hormones, such as cortisone or the Pill
- unhealthy 'hygienic' practices, such as the use of vaginal sprays or too frequent bubble baths
- stress.

This list is clearly not exhaustive, and in your own experience you may have noticed events which trigger vaginal infections. One triggering factor may be psychosomatic. Before the era of contraception, for example, women could more easily find an excuse to avoid making love when they didn't want to. Now, with the Pill, the IUD, and sterilization, the situation has become more difficult for those women who, for all kinds of reasons, do not dare tell their partners that they don't feel like making love. With a vaginal infection, on the other hand, penetration is out of the question . . . (although there are, of course, other possibilities!)

∽

Prevention of infections

- Wash your vulva with your hand rather than with a cloth, which is a perfect breeding ground for germs.
- Avoid douching in order not to eliminate the friendly bacteria which produce the protective acidity of the vagina.
- After using the toilet, wipe from the front to the back, and not the reverse, in order to avoid bringing germs from the rectum to the vagina.
- Don't use an alkaline soap (most soaps on the market are alkaline); it diminishes the acidity of the vagina. Or use an acid soap (which can be found in drug stores).
- Don't use so-called 'intimate' sprays which disrupt the vaginal *flora*. In this way we accomplish two things in one fell swoop: we prevent infection, and we refuse to lend support to a basically misogynous campaign that claims

that women smell. Have you ever heard it said that men's penises smell?

- Avoid pantihose and underclothes made of synthetic fibre. They prevent a proper circulation of air and create a hot-house climate whose warmth and humidity encourage the growth of germs which can affect the vagina.
- Wear underpants made of cotton which can be boiled or ironed at a high temperature.
- Avoid wearing tight pants. The friction leads to an inflammation of mucous membranes and from there to infection.
- Don't let a swimming suit dry on you. It can contain spores (germs at rest) which are only awaiting a favourable moment to increase in number. After swimming, wash the suit and let it dry well. This is especially important if you swim in swimming pools. The best thing is to swim in the nude, although this is unfortunately not often possible.

These are the precautions which a woman can take on her own. However, certain infections are transmitted by the partner through penetration. The partner therefore needs to observe good hygiene too. A man ought to wash his penis every day and just before sexual relations. The germs which can be found under the foreskin can, according to certain researchers, cause cancer of the cervix. Several American studies have shown that women who have sexual intercourse with circumcized men are less likely to have cancer of the cervix.

For lesbians, the risks of contamination are clearly less great, although a contact between the vaginal secretions of both women, via the fingers or the mouth, is possible. Good hygiene therefore includes nail care (nails should be short) and washing of hands.

కొ

Rapid recognition of infections

Most infections can be detected before symptoms such as discharge and itching occur. An examination of the vagina with the aid of a speculum will allow you to spot the first signs, if you are familiar with your vagina's normal state. For example, parts of the vagina or cervix may be redder than usual, or there may be small red spots on the cervix. With an infection, the colour, consistency and odour of the secretions change. It is easier to discern the colour of the secretions if (with a clean finger) you take a little discharge from the inner walls of the vagina and spread it on a glass slide.

Let's take a more detailed look at the most frequent agents of vulvar and vaginal burning:

- yeast
- trichomonas
- non-specific bacteria
- herpes
- condyloma
- chlamydia
- mycoplasma
- hemophilus (garderella, corynebacterium)
- streptococcus
- gonococcus
- treponema of syphilis.

We will conclude with chronic vaginal infections. AIDS will be addressed in Chapter 16.

৵

Yeast (or monilia *or* candida)

Yeast is a fungus whose spores are found just about everywhere – in swimming pools, sheets and beds. It is normally present in the vagina, and normally does not cause any trouble. However, if the ecological balance of the vagina is disturbed, it overgrows, especially in the deep part of the vagina and around the cervix.

The symptoms:

- Irritation, burning, itching of the vulva and the entrance to the vagina. Sometimes the vagina and the external parts are bright red, a sign of inflammation;
- White discharge, which smells of yeast and whose consistency resembles cottage cheese;
- Sometimes burning upon urination, and more frequent urination;
- If the vagina is examined with the help of a speculum, white patches can be seen. Underneath these, the walls of the vagina are red, rough, and irritated.

Examination: in order to be sure that it is yeast, a little of the discharge can be taken and spread on a microscopic slide. It is possible to see the fungus without colouring it, but in order to facilitate its detection amid the epithelial cells, KOH (hydroxide of potassium) can be used in place of physiological serum. KOH brings out the cells which appear like a clear carpet on which the darker filaments of yeast can be seen.

৵

What does modern western medicine propose?

Fungicide creams or suppositories with a nystatin base (such as Mycostatin†, or Monistat†), to be used locally. The treatment lasts 10 to 15 days, and it is important to finish the treatment completely, even if the symptoms have disappeared. These preparations can also be taken orally. This is recommended if the digestive system has also been invaded (sometimes with diarrhoea). This can be verified by examining the secretions collected from the rectum.

There are also other 'wide spectrum' preparations which attempt to treat several types of vaginal infections at the same time (Gynosterosan†). The disadvantage of these methods is that fungi become less and less sensitive to drugs which are taken too often (which leads to chronic states).

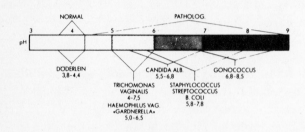

The alternative treatments

If the infection is detected early, adding lactic bacteria can be sufficient to restore a balance. *Active yogurt* (that is, non-pasteurized, containing live bacteria) can be used, or you may use one of the commercial preparations (*cultura lactobaccilli*) in tablet form. If there are several forms of lactic bacteria available in your area, you may want to try more than one if you have a reaction to one or the other (burning, allergy). Yogurt is of course the easiest tolerated, but its manipulation is a bit delicate. Yogurt can be introduced with a finger, speculum, or applicator intended for vaginal creams. When a speculum is used, put the speculum into place and then insert a spoon of yogurt. Remove the speculum, and *then* the spoon. Otherwise the yogurt stays in the speculum.

If the infection is more severe, you can begin with acidic vaginal douches (using vinegar or lemon juice, 2 teaspoons per bowl of water), twice a day for the first day or two, then moving on to the lactic bacteria treatment. Excessive douches should be avoided because you run the risk of eliminating lactic bacteria as well as the yeast fungi.

CAUTION: *vaginal douches are not recommended for pregnant women*.

Another possible treatment for those cases of tenacious yeast infections:

- vaginal douche of bicarbonate of soda (1 knifetip per bowl of water) mornings;
- garlic, morning and evening. Peel the clove of garlic without nicking it, otherwise it will burn you. You can put the clove in as it is, or wrapped in a strip of gauze or tied with a thread.
- lactic acid in the evening, in any form.
- the most active essential oils against yeast are: winter savory, lavender, palma rosa, melaleuca alternifolia.

Repeat all of this for 10 to 15 days.

Finally, gentian violet is also effective against yeast, although it stains. Gentian violet should not be used at more than 1 per cent per suppository, otherwise it burns.

To calm itching, you can use a cream or liquid form of camomile (see page 22, or tincture of calendula and golden-seal, diluted, as discussed on page 62) to rinse the vulva several times a day according to need.

Sexual relations with penetration are not advisable during treatment because they produce an additional irritation which is not only painful but can also lead to a flare-up of the infection.

Yeast infections are not dangerous, but they are troublesome because difficult to get rid of. A check-up should take place 4 to 7 days after the end of treatment to see if all signs of infection are gone. Sometimes there are no symptoms until the following menstrual period. The infection then takes off again because periods cause a change in the vaginal environment and a slight lowering of resistance. At the end of the bleeding, then, you may want to do a short preventive treatment.

Let's review the factors favouring an infection:

- antibiotics or other drugs prescribed for infection;
- pregnancy;
- taking the Pill or other hormones;
- diabetes or prediabetes.

Trichomonas

Trichomonas is a protozoa (cellular animal) which is present in the vagina, the intestines, the rectum of many women and men, and the urethra of many men – normally without causing problems. It is pear-shaped with 4 flagelles (kinds of threads) which enable it to move.

⤳

How do you catch trichomonas?

It is generally transmitted by:

- wet objects: swimming suits, underwear, towels and washcloths. Trichomonas can live outside the human body in a wet and warm environment;
- sexual contact;
- trich can spread from the rectum to the vagina if you wipe from the back to the front or through anal sexual relations followed by vaginal ones without proper washing in between.

Because trichomonas lives in a milieu which is less acid than the normal state of the vagina, everything which lowers this vaginal acidity permits a proliferation of trichomonas. This is the reason for a recurrence of trichomonas activity before menstrual bleeding.

ॐ

Symptoms

- itching and inflammation of the vulva and the entrance to the vagina;
- burning sensation at urination, although it is possible to have burning sensations at other times as well;
- greenish-yellow, evil-smelling discharge.

If the vagina is examined with the aid of a speculum, the beginnings of the infection can be seen. The vagina is redder than usual. There are sometimes small red spots the size of a pinhead on the walls of the vagina and on the cervix. The walls of the vagina can be painful, itchy, swollen or bleeding.

If trich is the only infecting organism, the discharge may be weak, frothy and yellow-green, but this is not necessarily true. If it is a mixed infection, which is more frequently the case, the discharge may be thick and white. If the discharge is very abundant, there can be an irritation on the inner thighs. Trich can spread to the urethra (urinary channel) and cause an infection of the urinary tract and burning.

Examination: To be completely sure that the infection is due to trichomonas, a little of the discharge may be taken and spread on a microscopic slide with a drop of physiological serum and looked at, enlarged to the 40th power (400 times). Trich is a little bit bigger than a white blood cell. If the slide is carried quickly to the microscope and the serum is lukewarm, trich can be seen to move between the cells and the white blood cells.

According to the statistics of the Polyclinic of Gynecology in Geneva, gonococcus was also found in 30 per cent of the cases of vaginal infections due to trichomonas (see below). It is therefore a good idea to also do a culture for gonococcus at the time of the diagnosis and to repeat it after the subsequent menstrual cycle.

꙰

What does modern western medicine propose?

The usual medical treatment is metronidazole (Flagyl†) or imidazole, in the form of tablets or vaginal suppositories. As trich is most often contracted through sexual contact, the partner should also be treated. Men do not generally show symptoms; they thus often do not know that they are harbouring trich until one of the women with whom they have sexual relations comes down with it.

There are contra-indications in the use of metronidazole:

- a disease of the blood, nervous system, or another infection at the same time;
- if you are pregnant or if you are breastfeeding, you should not take metronidazole orally (although you can use the vaginal suppositories) because it passes into the blood of the foetus or into the breast milk;
- if you drink alcohol during the treatment, you may be subject to nausea and vomiting as metronidazole blocks the digestive breaking down of alcohol. One glass thus has the effect of several;
- sometimes metronidazole causes dark urine.

Other side effects possible: nausea, diarrhoea, cramps, dizziness, metallic taste in the mouth, and dry mouth and vagina. Sometimes the treatment results in a yeast infection!

If you still have a discharge at the end of the treatment, you have perhaps picked up a fungus or contracted trich anew, or you have simply not been cured of the first infection. You must wait 4 to 6 weeks before starting treatment again because the metronidazole destroys white blood cells and your body has to replace them. Your doctor should do a white blood cell count before, during and after the second treatment. On the other hand, if you have contracted a fungus, you can be treated right away.

Thus metronidazole is not ideal. Furthermore, it is even suspected of still other misdeeds (for example, of having a possible involvement in cancer). So, until we know more about metronidazole, we prefer ornidazole, 500mg, 3 tablets in one dose, every evening.

ॐ

Alternative treatments

A clove of garlic, peeled as described earlier (page 71). Change the clove 2 to 3 times a day the first couple of days, then twice a day for a total of about 10 days. Since garlic also has a bactericide action, you should follow a garlic treatment by putting lactic bacteria in your vagina for several days.

Of course, this treatment only works for women. So if your partner is a man and he doesn't want to take chemical medication, he can experiment with garlic taken orally (1 pill 3 times a day) or capsules of garlic, 3 times a day. If 'garlic breath' is bothersome, sucking cumin will take it away. At this dose, garlic is a hypotensor, which brings us to discuss it in more detail.

Garlic (*Allium sativum*)
Part used: bulb, essence.
Properties: intestinal and pulmonary antiseptic, bacteriostatic and bactericide, stimulant, hypotensor, slows the pulse, anti-spasmodic, glandular equalizer, diuretic, activates digestion, and vermifuge. *In external use*: anti-parasitic, antalgic and tonic.
Indications: infectious diseases, diarrhoea, pulmonary illnesses (whooping cough), general weakness, arterial hypertension, hypercoagualability of the blood, renal lithiasis, gonorrhea, painful digestion, and parasites (ascaris, oxyures). *In external use*: corns, warts, wounds, wasp stings and insect bites. Garlic is *contra-indicated* by breastfeeding and congestive pulmonary symptoms: dry and strong cough, fever.

It is recommended to re-examine for infection after 10 days or 3 weeks of treatment.

Non-specific bacterial infections

These vaginal infections are caused by neither fungus nor by trichomonas. There are several species of bacteria which normally live in the vagina and are commonly called vaginal flora. The permanent secretion of the vagina is acidic (pH: 4.5), in part due to the lactic bacteria, also called Döderlein bacilles. It is this acidity which keeps the bacteria from proliferating.

As we noted at the beginning of the chapter, for an infection to break out, some assault must take place, such as an inflammation caused by penetration without sufficient lubrication, too-tight pants, or an iatrogenic attack: antibiotics, cortizones, or synthetic hormones which modify the acidity and favour microbiotic proliferation.

Having excluded venereal germs (such as gonococcus, chlamydia), we do not attempt to identify the microbes. For this reason, these infections are referred to as non-specific bacterial vaginal infections.

༴

Symptoms

- often the first sign is a need to urinate frequently and a sensation of burning during urination;
- pain in the lower back, cramps, swollen and painful glands, especially in the groin;
- the walls of the vagina are swollen and covered with a thick and viscous pus (most often made up of white blood cells which fight the infection, and of bacteria and dead cells). The pus can be white or yellow, sometimes having traces of blood.

- fairly severe vulvar itching.

If the infection is not treated rapidly, it can spread from the vagina to the urethra and the external labia. It can also reach the uterus and Fallopian tubes. This can cause sterility or a spontaneous abortion (miscarriage). Chronic infection can cause an abnormal increase in cells of the cervix and may be a factor favouring cancer through inflammation and irritation.

๛

What does modern western medicine propose?

Creams or vaginal suppositories based on sulphonamides or other antiseptics, even antibiotics: Sultrin† (sulphathiazole) 2 applications per day for 10 days, chloroquinaldol, 1 suppository per day for 10 days, Terramycin†, 1 suppository per day for 7 days ... These are always followed up by a series of lactic bacteria.

These treatments may be effective for an acute infection, but we would not recommend them in cases of chronic infection because they diminish resistance. We would also not recommend the use of vaginal disinfectants (such as Viranol†) as a preventive measure because they destroy the balance of protective flora.

๛

Alternative treatments

At the first sign of an infection, begin with acidic douches (lemon juice or vinegar, preferably home-made vinegar – without colouring or conserving agent! – diluted with water), twice a day for 10 days, then switch to a treatment of lactic bacteria.

However, phytotherapy has a lot more to offer in this area with the fantastic anti-microbiotic action of herbs and in particular of essential oils (aromatherapy).

These methods are equally useful for the yeast and trichomonas infections discussed above, but we will discuss them only in the section on bacterial infections.

But let's look first of all at a few general points, including the question of *when to start treatment*.

When a non-specific bacteria infection is involved, a microscopic examination of the discharge will show a considerable number of flora (which is not a criterion sufficient in itself), and an elevated number of white blood cells, signalling an inflammation.

It is normal to have some white blood cells before menstrual bleeding and at ovulation, and a woman with an IUD almost always has them because the foreign body can cause a chronic inflammation. It is important not to rely on the microscope alone, but to pay attention to the signs the woman may be feeling. Even in the absence of an infection, it can still be judicious to do a *treatment*: before placing an IUD, for example, or at the time of an abnormal cervical smear, to be redone under better conditions.

To stimulate the local circulation, you can try cold sitz-baths or exercises which contract and relax the perineal muscles (like in childbirth preparation). After a while, you even learn how to contract the vagina and anus separately without anybody noticing anything – in a bus, for example.

৵

What herbs can be used?

Goldenseal (*Hydrastis canadensis*)
Part used: rhizome.
Properties: tonic, pelvic vaso-constrictor, hemostatic, anti-sudorific, aids secretion of bile.
Indications: haemorrhoids, varicose veins, uterine haemorrhage,

congested state of the body and cervix of the uterus, constipation of the biliaries, leg ulcer, lowered resistance to infection.

Decoction of the root: 60g herb per litre liquid, 2 to 3 cups a day.

Tincture: 30 to 120 drops a day, taken orally or diluted in water in vaginal douches. This herb associates well with one of the following two herbs:

Calendula (*Calendula officinalis*)

Part used: flower.

Properties: regulator of periods and calmer of their pain, depurative, diuretic, hypotensor through peripheral vaso-dilation, stimulant, anti-cancer, antiseptic and aid in formation of scar tissue, excellent remedy for wounds.

Indications: scanty menstrual flow, painful periods, hepatic congestion, gastric ulcer. *In external use*: ulcers, fissures, wounds, boils, burns.

Infusion: 1 teaspoon per cup liquid.

Tincture: 60 to 120 drops per day.

In external use: tincture diluted to 10 drops per cup liquid, 1 teaspoon for 1 litre or calendula in a cream form.

Its name derives from the 'herb which comforts' of the ancients who were familiar with comfrey's various powers, one of which is to speed the healing of fractures.

Comfrey (*Symphytum officinale*)

Part used: root.

Properties: softener, astringent, aids healing of wounds.

Indications: enteritis, diarrhoea, ulcers, bronchitis, white vaginal discharge and genital infections. *In external use*: wounds, burns, leg ulcers, cracked nipples, anal fissures.

Maceration of the root: 150g per litre water. Boil and let macerate. Drink within 24 hours.

Tincture: 5 to 20 drops, 3 to 4 times a day.

In homoeopathy, *symphytum* is indicated in trauma to the bone and periosteum (fracture) and to the eye (with the exception of a black eye).

Reserve group in tincture: mallow, loosestrife, marshmallow, oak, water-lily, fenugreek.

There are more than 40 herbs noted for their antiseptic effect. We will cite here only the most frequently used: oregano, savory, clove, cinnamon, eucalyptus, geranium, cajeput, pine, lavender, thyme, sage and thuja.

꒚

Essential oils

One of the most practical ways to use herbs in treating infections is in the form of *essential oils* or of essences, usually obtained by distilling the herbs and mixing the distillation with oil and alcohol. Essential oils (EO) can be used either locally or internally (see Appendix 2).

The extraordinary contribution of aromatherapy (treatment by essences of herbs) in vaginitis is that herbs have a powerful bactericide effect which does not diminish over time. It is for this reason that they have been used for thousands of years (the same, we might point out, cannot be said for antibiotics). It also offers the possibility of an individualized treatment.

The aromatogram

This involves making a culture from the vaginal discharge and, after 24 hours, exposing these germs to a drop of each EO (on a piece of saturated blotting paper), to see which are the best killers. It is a procedure similar to an anti-biogram, but with EO used in the place of antibiotics.

Of course, the results are valid for a limited time only (germs change, as do the women who carry them). Furthermore, to be sure of effectiveness, you should use exactly the same EO, not only from the same plant, but one from the same area and same lot.

By making a culture not only of the vaginal discharge, but also of an anal and throat swab, and in choosing the herbs which have the most effect on all three samples, we can discern the herbs which treat the 'ground'. That is, herbs which act against the woman's other weaknesses and which strengthen the organism as a whole. For example, eucalyptus in a prediabetic woman or juniper or geranium for an arthritic woman.

According to a study carried out by Dr Belaiche on the antiseptic power of EO on 12 different pathogens, essences which are fungicides have about the same effect as those essences which are bactericides. A useful point to know. However, if you have not done an aromatogram, you should not expect a guaranteed result, even from oregano and clove, which have been the most consistently effective in the women we have treated. After all, an aromatogram is a more precise 'picture' of a specific woman's state at a specific moment. Since then great progress has been made in aromatherapy with the work of P. Collin and P. Franchomme to clarify the *chemotypes*. There are for example different sorts of thyme (thymus vulgaris), one with thymol (phenols), the other with tuyanol (alcohols). There are also different sorts of melaleuca: the m. leucadendron: cajeput, le m. alternifolia (alcohols) and the m. pentanerve or quinquinervia: niaouli (oxides). It is easy to understand that these plants will have different properties and that if they grow in different regions they will be used differently. This work has clarified the need to use the botanic names with the chemotype (CTEO: chemotyped essential oil). If an essential oil has been chosen after an aromatogram, the prescription should also mention the batch number and the producer so that the pharmacist will use the same oil as the one tested in the lab – this is for scientific precision!

Classification by their principal components is as follows: phenols, alcohols, ethers, esters, oxides, terpenes and cetones are going from the most tonifying (positive electric class) to the most sedative or dispersing (negative electric class). The anti-microbial activity is directly proportionate to the degree of positive ionization. One should, however, be careful in the use of phenols because of their toxicity on the mucous membrane, the liver and immuno-depressive effect after 8–10 days of use.

But let's take a look at a few herbs in more detail, looking perhaps for 'ground' indications. We have already see *sage* in irregular periods and amenorrhea, *lavender* in amenorrhea, and in bleeding *thuja, clove, cinnamon* and *geranium*.

Marjoram (*Origanum vulgare*)

Properties: sedative, anti-spasmodic, digestive, expectorant, antiseptic of the respiratory passages, emmenagogue.

Indications: lack of appetite, slow digestion, chronic bronchitis and irritated cough, asthma, amenorrhea.

Infusion: 1 teaspoon per cup liquid.

EO: 3 to 5 drops, 2 to 4 times a day (see below for the excipient).

This dose is identical for the following 4 herbs.

Winter savory (*Satureia montana*)

Properties: digestive, stimulant (of the intellect), anti-spasmodic, antiseptic, in particular anti-fungicide.

Indications: difficult digestion, intellectual and sexual fatigue, nervous gastric pain, intestinal fermentation, intestinal parasites, asthma, bronchitis.

Eucalyptus (*Eucalyptus globulus*)

Properties: antiseptic, especially of respiratory and urinary passages, hypoglycimiant, vermifuge, antirheumatic. *In external use*: bactericide, parasiticide, mosquito repellant.

Indications: bronchitis, flu, tuberculosis, colibacillosis, diabetes, rheumatism, intestinal parasites (ascaris, oxyures), and migraine.

The *eucalyptus raviata* is used in EO against herpes. In strong doses, this essence can provoke headaches, a kind of drunkenness, and prostration.

Cajeput (*Malaleuca leucadendron*)

Properties: antiseptic, anti-spasmodic, anti-neuralgia, vermifuge.

Indications: enteritis, cystitis, chronic pulmonary ailments, gastric spasm, asthma, nervous vomiting, painful periods, rheumatism and intestinal parasites.

The niaouli (melaleuca quinquinervia) is a particularly interesting species for its hormonal regulation action on the hypophyse-ovary axe and against anti-herpes. It is used to stimulate the cortico-adrenals and in the dysplasia and condyloma (oxides group). The melaleuca alternifolia (alcohol group) is more active as an anti-microbial.

Pine (*Pinus sylvestris*)
Properties: antiseptic of respiratory passage, flu, urinary ailments, cholecystitis, biliary lithiasis, impotence and intestinal pain.

CAUTION: *those EOs which are rich in phenols – clove* (Eugenia caryophyllata), *oregano* (Origanum compactum), *parsley* (Petroselinum sativum), *savory* (Satureia montana), *and thyme* (Thymus vulgaris) – *can burn the mucous membrane*. In our experience, we have had no complaints because the EOs were diluted to less than 1 per cent.

༈

How to use these tinctures and essential oils (see also Appendix 2)
Example of a liquid for use in vaginal douche

tincture goldenseal
tincture calendula   } aa qsp 60ml
kalium bichromicum 3X

Dilute one teaspoon of this liquid in one litre water. For use in 2 to 3 irrigations per day.

Bichromate of potassium (*Kalium bichromicum*) is used in

homoeopathy for its action on mucus membranes in the presence of an inflammation with abundant thick yellow-green mucus.

∽

Example of a vaginal suppository: see page 104

If you want to take EO orally, as part of a general treatment, some precautions are necessary because essential oils can be damaging to the gastric mucus and cause burns (even ulcers).

CAUTION: *do not exceed the given quantities.* When it says 3 drops, it doesn't mean 5. Essential oils are to be taken after meals. The following is an example of one of the best ways to mix them.

EO 1		
EO 2	according to the aromatogram[1]	aa 1g
EO 3		
alcohol 94%		25g
glycerine 98%		10g

Take 25 drops, 3 to 4 times a day after meals.

CAUTION: EOs which are rich in phenols (see page 83) have an immuno-stimulating effect the first 6 days, and an immuno-suppressant effect beyond 8 days. They should therefore be used only in a treatment of 'attack', for example, before receiving the results of the aromatogram.

Other naturopaths prescribe EOs in an elixir of papain. Papain is indeed a powerful digestive, but an elixir is made with a lot of sugar and, what's more, with a preserving agent. For this reason, we no longer use it.

---

[1] If cinnamon (bark) is prominent in the aromatogram, it is preferable to use it alone because its effect is diminished rather than enhanced by the presence of other herbs.

Essential oils can also be taken in the form of micro-douches or creams. For other formulas, see Appendix 1 on 'phyto' definitions and formulas.

Chinese medicine uses:

Sunflower
Part used: flowers.
Properties: for westerners: febrifuge.
Indications: fever, malaria, spleen ailments (homoeopathy).
Dosage for westerners: tincture at ⅒ of flowers, 25 drops, 3 times a day.
Dosage for Chinese: decoction of 15g of flowers with 30g of brown (!) sugar in cases of white vaginal discharge with pale face, cold hands and feet, backache and weakness in the legs, fatigue, flat taste in mouth, clear and abundant urine, and weak and deficient pulse.

It should be noted that Chinese medicine also uses vinegar in cases of vaginitis (along with other herbs with which we here in the west are not familiar) and that in non-venereal vaginitis, the differentiation between germs is not important.

Herpes

Herpes is an infectious disease caused by a virus, herpes simplex, of which there are two types (I and II). Herpes simplex I is responsible for what is commonly called the 'cold sore' which appears in the area of the mouth or elsewhere on the skin; herpes simplex II, for a vaginal infection which is most often seen on the vulva. The widespread incidence of herpes today underscores the importance of 'ground' in one's receptiveness to this virus. There are people who are carriers of herpes but who themselves do not have it.

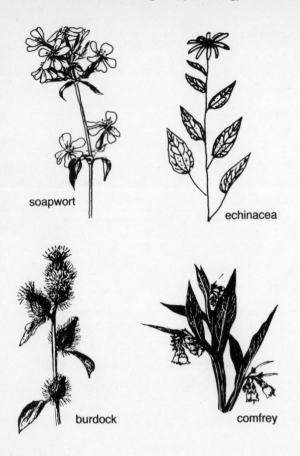

soapwort

echinacea

burdock

comfrey

The symptoms

- The first sign is an inflamed and sensitive area, possibly accompanied by swollen and painful glands.
- The next sign is the appearance of small white blisters which open into painful sores. The sores heal spontaneously in one to two weeks.

Vaginal herpes is transmitted through sexual contact. The actively contagious sore is unfortunately not always visible; it can be located within the penis or deep within the vagina.

Herpes simplex has a cousin, herpes zoster, the cause of zona, a phenomenon quite similar to herpes simplex but in which the blisters appear in a belt-like formation or along the path of a sensitive nerve.

⨍

Risks

In themselves the sores present a risk of secondary infection. In addition, if a baby is contaminated at birth by vaginal herpes, s/he risks cerebral lesions. Active vaginal herpes is therefore widely recognized as an indication for a cesarean.

⨍

What does modern western medicine propose?

Modern western medicine has in fact nothing concrete to propose. Local analgesics in cream form can be used for the discomfort (for example, Nupercainal†), just as antibiotic creams can be used to fight a bacterial secondary infection. But nothing is used to *treat* herpes itself, except perhaps the new anti-viral creams (Viru-merz†, Virunguent†, Acyclovir†, Zovirax†) which are effective in stopping an outbreak of herpes, especially if employed within the first few days of an attack. However, they have no fundamental effect and do not prevent recurrences. Research is presently underway to develop a vaccine. Using this contagious illness as part of a campaign against 'sexual promiscuity' and homosexuality in order to 'strengthen the family', the New Right in the United States has its own proposal: 'remain a virgin until marriage, marry a virgin, and remain "faithful".'

ཟ

What are the alternatives?

Here again we cannot help being enthusiastic about phyto-therapy. For while modern western remedies seem unable to reinforce immunities in the body, natural medicines are much more successful.

In general: since herpes is associated with *stress*, among other things, *rest* is helpful. In diet, one should avoid coffee and other stimulants (tea, nicotine, drugs) as well as *sugar*, since these diminish resistance to infections (for more on diet and immunity, see chapter 15). For local applications, camomile or calendula can be used in sitz-baths. This helps clean the sores, but relieves pain only minimally. *Dwarf Nettle* (*urtica urens*) diluted to 10 per cent or less with calendula and an excipient relieves more effectively.

The most active EOs against herpes are: niaouli (m. quinqui-nervia), ravensare aromatica and eucalyptus raviata. They are all well tolerated in ovulas, even at more than 10 per cent.

ཟ

Specific treatments

We owe the use of echinacea as a treatment for herpes to a worker at the Women's Health Service in Sante Fe, New Mexico, and to a herbalist working in the same city.

Echinacea (*Echinacea augustifolia L.*)
This is a hardy plant which can reach 60 to 90cm in height. It has a single stalk covered with coarse hair. The leaves are thick, rough, and hairy with three strong veins. It has a single flower which blooms from July to October and its colour varies from pale pink to light purple.

Part used: dried rhizome, root.

Properties: sudorific, increases salivary secretions.

Indications: Echinacea is useful in all diseases due to impurities of the blood. Naturopaths have always maintained that echinacea is the ideal vegetable anti-toxin, and modern western medicine has always denied or ignored it. For native Americans, echinacea has an honourable place in the treatment of infections, different forms of septicaemias, blood poisoning (toxins which the body is unable to eliminate), typhoid fever, abscesses, salpingitis, and fevers due to internal or external infections. The Sioux Indians use the freshly ground root against rabies, snake bites and skin infections.

Preparation and dosage: Soak the root (cut into pieces) in a cup of boiling water for half an hour. Filter and take one tablespoon 3 to 6 times a day. This liquid can also be applied to the skin.

Tincture: 5 to 200 drops at a time, depending on whom you consult.

This plant is not toxic in large quantities, although it is known to cause abundant salivation.

Homoeopathy uses a tincture of the entire plant, freshly diluted or dynamized for appendicitis, rabid animal bites, blood poisoning, diphtheria, gangrene, scarlet fever, septicaemia, snake bites, syphilis, typhoid and the effects of vaccinations.

For the Russians (for a change from the Chinese), echinacea is an antiseptic for internal as well as external use. In internal use, it reduces pain and strengthens the immunological potential of the blood to resist infection and the spread of disease.

Dosage of the Women's Health Center: At the first sign of a herpes attack, take 25 drops of tincture of echinacea in a little water every 2 hours for 6 to 8 hours. Then 4 times a day through the duration of the attack. Taken early, echinacea prevents or shortens the outbreak. Herpes rarely recurs more than once after a treatment of echinacea.

In phytotherapy, there are several other plants known to be effective.

Burdock (*Arctium lappa*)

Part used: root.

Properties: depurative, sudorific, antiseptic (in particular, staphylococcus and gram positive germs), stimulates hepato-biliary secretions, diuretic.

Indications: syphilis (?), boils, eczema, impetigo, herpes, rheumatism, cough.

Decoction: 15 to 60g per litre liquid for local use (as a compress) or orally.

Tincture: 6 to 25 drops at a time, 3 times a day.

Boxwood (*Buxus sempervirens*)

Part used: leaf, peel of root.

Properties: depurative, sudorific, laxative, stimulates hepato-biliary secretions, disinfectant and vulnerary, febrifuge.

Indications: biliary insufficiency or infection, fever, rheumatism, gout, syphilis (?), atonic and infected wounds.

Infusion: 1 teaspoon per liquid.

Decoction: 40g per litre liquid, 3 cups per day in poultice or gargle form.

Tincture: 25 drops before the two main meals.

Soapwort (*Saponaria officinalis*)

Part used: entire plant.

Properties: depurative, diuretic, sudorific, increases hepato-biliary secretions, vermifuge.

Indications: rheumatism, infected urinary and hepatic passages, fatigue, fever, syphilis (?), cancer (?). *In external use*: herpes and diverse dermatoses.

Decoction: 50g per litre liquid, 2 cups a day. (Don't let the plant macerate as this can be toxic.) Can be used as poultice or gargle.

Tincture: 25 drops, twice a day.

Another plant known to both Chinese medicine and that of Central America:

Sarsaparilla (*Smilax aspera*) (Spanish: *zarzaparilla*)
Part used: root.
Properties: Progesterone-like, diuretic, depurative, cleans the blood of impurities, stimulates the immunity.
Indications: intoxication, rheumatism, dermatose, herpes.
Decoction: a large piece of root (crushed) per cup liquid, 2 to 3 cups a day.
Tincture: 2–4g a day.

If these methods fail, a 'ground' treatment (homoeopathy, acupuncture, osteopathy) should be considered.

Condyloma

Condyloma is a kind of wart which has the disagreeable idea of growing on the vulva, the vagina or the cervix. When they are microscopic, condylomas do not cause any symptoms, but can affect pap smear results. When they become visible to the naked eye, as white and shiny ridges, they can cause a severe burning sensation. Condyloma is transmitted through sexual contact, but 'ground' is an important factor in whether one catches them or not.

ᴣ

What does modern western medicine propose?

About the same technique as for other warts: burning, freezing, excision: electrocoagulation, cryotherapy (under general anaesthesia, if necessary) laser or surgery. As is true of treatment of other warts, the results are very uneven, and the warts frequently reappear.

ॐ

What are the alternatives?

Tincture of thuja, one or two applications per day. Mandrake in a tincture of 25 per cent gum bezoin, twice a week, rinsing after 15 to 20 minutes with an infusion of camomile or diluted tincture of calendula (otherwise it burns!)

Thuja can also be taken orally: in tincture form, 10 drops twice a day, or in homoeopathy: thuja 4 CH, 2 granules, 3 times a day.

EO of niaouli is very effective in cases of cervical condyloma.

EO niaouli
EO mugwort   } aa 10% in hazel oil
3 applications a day.

This is for the visible condyloma or shiny ridges. For the atypic of plain one, use EO niaouli (*m. quinquinervia*) 3–4 drops per ovula of 3g, one ovula at night, even during periods. If there is no result after a month, increase to 12 drops for a prolonged treatment.

Finally, colchicum tincture is another possibility which quite simply inhibits cellular division, for local use only. CAUTION! *Colchicum is very toxic when taken orally!* Colchicum is the basis of the first anti-mitotics (drugs which hinder cellular proliferation, for example, in cancer treatment).

Mandrake (*Podophyllum peltatum*)
Part used: root.
Properties: cholagogue, drastic purgative.
Indications: chronic constipation (for example, in paralytics), biliary lithiasis.
In external use: condylomas.

Where these treatments do not work, a treatment of 'ground' – acupuncture or homoeopathy – needs to be undertaken.

Before addressing the traditional venereal agents (gonorrhea and syphilis), let's take a look at a few 'new' germs.

Chlamydia

Chlamydia has only been identified and studied as a bacteria since the 1970s. Before this time, it was believed that chlamys was a virus because of its size and its habit of living in cells. However, it is indeed a bacteria: gram-negative, oval-round, and three times smaller than streptococcus.

According to American sources, it seems that young women and women on the Pill are those more frequently attacked by chlamys.

✥

The signs

Ten to 20 days after contact, cervicitis or urethritis most often appears. Untreated, 20 per cent of the infections develop into a pelvic infection. The pelvic infection is less violent than that of gonorrhea, the fever may be moderate, painful possibly only during intercourse. Swelling is bilateral.

Chlamydia can also be responsible for perihepatitis. That is, an infection of the capsule of the liver causing fever, painful percussion of the liver, and grating at auscultation (as in pericarditis). Hepatic tests are not necessarily affected.

In men, there is a discharge from the penis, which is clearer than that of gonorrhea.

Women and men can have an infection of the rectum: painful bowel movements, burning of the rectum, bleeding or pus. They can also have conjunctivitis.

In pregnant women, the risk for the baby is conjunctivitis and pneumonia (10–20 per cent of exposed babies, according to the sources). Most studies on chlamydia are on this topic.

Much more will have to be written about chlamydia, which,

as we've noted, has only recently been discovered, before we know its true virulence.

꒰ꇙ꒱

What does modern western medicine propose?

As chlamydia is often associated with gonorrhea, treatment is often a derivative of tetracycline (Vibramycin† or Erythromycin†), 200mg the first day, then 100mg for 10 days.

Locally, Fungizone† can be used (tetracycline-amphotericine, a wide-range antibiotic used in treatment of: yeast, mixed bacteria, trichomonas, mycoplasm, chlamydia).

꒰ꇙ꒱

What are the alternatives?

When antibiotics do not work anymore, one can use *EO thyme thuyanol-4* (alcohol), which has no hepato-toxicity and is an immuno-stimulant. Take orally 1.5g in 10ml of alcohol/glycerine mixture, 3 times a day, for 3 months or 0.3g CTEO in an ovula of 3g, one a night for 3–6 months.

Note: I'm insisting on the chemotype thuyanol-4 because the thymus vulg. with thymol (phenols) would burn in local use and couldn't be used orally for more than 10 days because of its toxicity.

༄

Mycoplasma

Mycoplasma is a very small germ-like ureaplasma which has been cultured for less time than chlamydia and which is also transmitted by sexual contact.

Signs: nothing, or vaginitis (in men, urethritis or prostatitis), burning sensation at urination, bartholinitis, (see page 119), cervicitis, a pelvic infection (endometritis, salpingitis), fever after childbirth or abortion.

It is thought by some that mycoplasma may be responsible for sterility, but this has not been proven. Others describe it as being implicated in Reiter's syndrome (which begins with abdominal pain and diarrhoea, followed by urethritis or non-gonorrheal conjunctivitis, then a painful and feverish polyarthritis which evolves by stages). Despite this possible connection of great interest to university medicine, it all boils down to a lot of supposition on the role of mycoplasma, especially since it is possible that it doesn't cause *anything*, and that it exists as part of the flora in a 'state of peace' with the host!

As mycoplasma is often associated with gonorrhea, treatment for the moment is tetracycline (Vibramycin†) from 1 to 3 weeks (average being 2 weeks), treating the partner(s) as well.

It is here that the discussion begins.

When mycoplasma is associated with gonorrhea, everyone agrees on an antibiotic treatment. On the other hand, if we indiscriminately use antibiotics in all types of vaginitis, and even without signs, we will quickly create resistant strains. Since this is perhaps not the best trade-off, it becomes tempting to study other possible ways of dealing with these situations. Aromatherapy and phytotherapy, certainly, have a lot to offer in this area (see section on 'Non-specific bacterial infections', page 76).

To add a practical note, to get the result of a mycoplasma culture, as well as a gene culture takes 24 hours. In an acute case the woman would have already started treatment.

Hemophilus Gardnerella or Cornyebactirium

Hemophilus is another of those germs which has had the honour of being entered into the classification of 'venereal', that is, it can be transmitted by sexual contact.

Shaped like a pin with a head, this germ can be both aerobic and anaerobic (able to live with or without air), and is recognizable by its manner of 'dotting' cells.

Hemophilus causes a very clear, grey discharge. Men are rarely attacked by hemophilus, and in women it is hardly worse than vaginitis, except after obstetrical trauma (cesarean and puerperal fever). (This is not to suggest that vaginitis is not unpleasant!)

Certain authors have none the less distinguished it from the other non-specific bacterial infections because there is a high rate of re-infection in women whose partners are not treated.

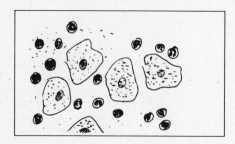

In the presence of garderella, secretions on a slide in contact with a KOH drop will release a characteristic rotten-fish smell.

ॐ

What does modern western medicine propose?

Metronidazole (Flagyl†), at first (see trichomonas), and afterward, Vibramycine†, 250mg for 4 days, ampicillin, 500mg 4 times a day for 7 days, and sulphidamides for local use for 15 days.

ॐ

What do we propose?

We keep the Flagyl† for local use for women who prefer allopathic treatments, and otherwise use lively lactobacilles
powder (Ribolac†) in a lactic acid cream. If it doesn't work
then consider treating the partner's classically and then use the
same methods as for chronic vaginal infections.

Streptococcus (beta) hemolytic, group B

Here we enter into a statistical dispute: *are* there more group B
streptococcus in male patients seeking treatment for 'venereal'
diseases (possibly associated with gonorrhea) than in control
groups (the same number of supposedly healthy persons)? It
is, in any case, a germ less pathological than the preceding
ones.

Streptococcus entered the group of sexually transmitted
diseases by the side door. More descriptions are of isolated
cases than of major trends.

Modern western medicine proposes none the less: 10 days
of ampicillin 3g a day, or amoxicillin, 750mg 3 times a day for
10 days.

Systematic use of antibiotics in even benign infections inevi-
tably leads to a mutation of germs, which become antibiotic-
resistant. Instead, we need to find ways of becoming more
resistant to the bacteria and other microbes with which we
share this planet and which are useful to us in the decomposi-
tion of waste. See also methods under non-specific bacterial
vaginal infections or chronical vaginal infections, pages 76,
102.

Let's take a brief look at two diseases which are definitely
venereal:

Gonorrhea

Gonorrhea is caused by a bacteria whose form is that of a coffee bean, naesseria gonorrhea or gonococcus.

In men, gonorrhea makes its presence known in the early stages: discharge from the penis or burning at urination. In women, on the other hand, the early stages are without symptoms. Occasionally, women will have signs within 2 days to 3 weeks after exposure: yellow-green discharge, itching, or urinary burning – all of which may easily pass for an ordinary vaginitis or cervicitis.

When the infection reaches the uterus and Fallopian tubes, the woman may feel pain in her lower abdomen or in her back. Sometimes, there is also fever and vomiting; periods become irregular.

Untreated, gonorrhea doesn't stop here. It can cause arthritis, meningitis, inflammation of the heart valves, blindness, sterility and even death.

An infant can contract gonorrhea in its eyes during its passage through the vagina at birth. Thus it is standard practice in hospitals to put drops of silver nitrate in the eyes of all newborns, as a preventive measure.

TEST: cultures must be done from secretions taken from the cervix, urinary meatus, and throat, areas most susceptible to gonorrhea (the same is true for chlamydia and mycoplasma, by the way). If the test is being performed as a means of checking on the effectiveness of a treatment, or in the absence of signs, it is preferable to do the test at the end of menstrual bleeding. The germ can be coloured with methylene blue or gram colour. Gonococcus resembles a coffee bean. It can be found in white blood cells and its surrounding bacterial flora are generally poor.

৵

What does modern western medicine propose?

Penicillin and its derivatives, tetracyclines. In early stages, or for women having a partner with a positive culture, spectinomycin (Trobicin†) can be used intramuscularly: 2g for men, 4g for women; or amoxycillin: 4 tablets of 750mg in one dose.

Once removed from its environment, gonococcus is a fragile germ. It is therefore recommended to do a second culture to verify treatment.

৵

What are the alternatives?

As the readers will have come to realize during the preceding chapters, we are not great adventurers in alternative treatment for gonorrhea – we too propose antibiotics! The two instances where we might attempt another method would be in the case of a gonorrhea which was chronic and resistant to conventional treatment, or in the case of vaginitis in women in good general condition and firmly set against antibiotics (we can tell you that this is rare where gonorrhea is involved!).

It might be interesting to mention, however, a few herbs which – according to knowledge which dates from well before the epoch of antibiotics – are reputed to have an anti-gonorrhea action, but which we ourselves have never used.

In tincture: uva ursi (*Arbutus uva ursi*), shepherd's purse (*Capsella bursa pastoris*), and *Piper methysticum*.
In essential oil: sandalwood (*Santalum spicatum*), garlic, and juniper (*Juniperus communis*).

These herbs are cited in other chapters, which makes them

even more valuable. It should be mentioned, too, that gonorrhea and syphilis, when cut down by antibiotics, can cause problems of elimination, which are expressed as warts. At the Women's Health Center, we 'drain' these antibiotics through homoeopathy (that is, we give the antibiotic again, in minute homoeopathic doses, in order to break up the congestion created by suppressing the symptoms).

Syphilis

Syphilis is a systemic infectious disease caused by the treponema (pallidum). The infection directly affects the entire body through the circulation of the blood. It can be hereditary or acquired. In the latter case, the infection is transmitted sexually, through a mucous membrane or a cutaneous lesion (chancre).

Clinically, the disease evolves in three phases of increasing severity if left untreated (there are few spontaneous recoveries from syphilis).

$\sim$

Primary syphilis

The *period of incubation* varies from 1 to 12 weeks, but generally lasts 3 to 4 weeks from the contaminating contact. A chancre (sore) appears. That is, a spot which reddens and then ulcerates. Sometimes there may be several chancres. Chancres can generally be found in the genital area, but they can also appear in or around the mouth, on the fingers, etc. The chancre does not bleed and is not painful, but the fluid which seeps from it is highly contagious.

At this stage, some of the fluid can be collected and examined under a microscope in order to find the treponemas on a black background. At this time, the local lymphatic glands will be enlarged and soft, but not painful. This phase lasts several weeks and ends with the healing of the chancre.

The *secondary phase* begins about 6 to 8 weeks after the beginning of the infection, and manifests itself through all kinds of symptoms, especially cutaneous ones. (Since venereal diseases imitate* all kinds of skin problems, they are in general diagnosed and connected with dermatology!)

The very variable cutaneous lesions of syphilis may take the form of a 'roseole' (small red spots) on the thorax and the back, or brick-red eruptions on the trunk, the limbs, the palms of the hand, the face, or the crook of the arm. White spots may appear on the tongue and the inner cheeks. The genital mucous membranes may be the site of escrescences called condylomas (to be distinguished from common acuminated condylomas). There is in particular an enlargement of all the lymphatic glands and of the liver and spleen. The person may experience fatigue, aches, pain in the bones, stiff neck, or loss of hair. Of course, at this stage, all the lesions are contagious, but a diagnosis is made on the basis of blood serum tests, specific to syphilis, which measure the immunity of the body.

There is generally a spontaneous remission of these symptoms, with possible relapses. Next is a *latent phase*, which may last from two to twenty years, during which the person appears completely normal.

This latent phase is divided into early latency (less than four years after infection), during which the person is potentially contagious and can suffer a relapse of secondary syphilis; and late latency (more than four years), which is not contagious (except for a foetus).

Tertiary syphilis presents itself in 50 to 75 per cent of untreated cases, through deeper and more destructive lesions of the skin, bones, veins, nervous system, and cardio-vascular system which we are not going to describe in detail here. This stage is that of a chronic disease which generally leads to death.

Congenital syphilis. Syphilis is transmitted from the mother to the foetus through the placenta, after the fourth month of pregnancy. It can, however, be detected and treated in time. The greatest risk for the foetus is when the infection is recent. Serious defects may be present at birth (deformation of the skin, bones, or teeth, meningitis, paralysis, mental retardation, etc.), or the child may slowly develop the symptoms of tertiary syphilis throughout his or her life.

The treatment of all the stages is intra-muscular penicillin G. For the later stages, treatment is carried out over several weeks. In primary syphilis, one treatment may be sufficient.

As mentioned in our discussion on gonorrhea, a syphilitic infection blocked by antibiotics constitutes a favourable 'ground' for other health problems. It is one of three basic 'grounds' in homoeopathy, known by the name of huès (meaning source of illness). It is necessary, therefore, after a treatment of antibiotics, to do a homoeopathic treatment which cleanses the body of the traces of the syphilitic infection.

Again, we have no experience with herbal treatment of syphilis, but there are those who cite sassafras, lemon, boxwood, burdock, soapwort and pansy.

AIDS will be addressed in Chapter 16.

Chronic vaginal infections

These lead us into yet another section where phyto-aromatherapy has a lot to offer, whether the agent be yeast, trichomonas or bacteria.

The first step in the treatment of chronic vaginal infections is a review of the elements of hygiene and prevention cited at the beginning of the chapter (page 66), adding a piece of advice for women subject to chronic vaginal infection: give up using (menstrual) tampons, a perfect haven for germs. Diet is another important consideration, as it can help or hinder the reinforcement of resistance to infection. Pay special attention to alcohol, drugs and medication (including the Pill).

ॐ

What has modern western medicine to offer?

It has nothing in particular to offer, other than to repeat treatments in the case of yeast, to prescribe that fungicides be taken orally instead of applied locally, or, as a preventive measure, to use local disinfectants after each menstrual period.

As the reader will have realized, we think that this approach runs the risk of making a chronic situation worse rather than better.

ॐ

What are the alternatives?

Below is the therapeutic outline *we* propose:

(a) *Selection of trace-elements*
Copper may be used in practically all infectious situations, but it may be more useful to determine into which *diathesis* the woman falls. This is essentially seen from her daily cycle of energy (rhythm of rise and fall in energy level, sudden drops in energy, whether she gains a 'second wind' in the evening, insomnia . . .) and of her behaviour. It is preferable to use a trace-element corresponding to a diathesis, if one is clear. Otherwise, copper can be used, or the idea of trace-elements should be abandoned (see page 215 or, better still, References).

(b) *Hepato-renal draining*
To aid the elimination of toxins from the body and fight against constipation, we propose the following preparation:

tincture artichoke
tincture boldo   } aa 5g
tincture fumitory
tincture condurango
tincture turmeric   } aa 3g
tincture rosemary
tincture olea europea,
   diluted to 10% qsp
   120ml

50 to 80 drops before eating, or 40 drops before the two main meals.

(olea europea = olive oil!)

(c) *General preparation*

tincture sweet briar
tincture blackcurrant
tincture raspberry   } aa qsq 100ml
tincture shave grass
tincture pansy

50 to 80 drops, 3 times a day.

(d) *And according to the aromatogram*

In suppository form for local use:

EO 1
EO 2   } 1 drop
EO 3
tincture marigold
tincture goldenseal } aa 0.03g
green clay   aa 0.075g
excipient   qsp 1 ovule of 3g

1 suppository each evening.

EO niaouli
EO myrtus communis   } aa qsp 0.3g
EO salvia sclarea
exipient   qsp 1 ovule of 3g

1 at night.

Orally:

EO 1
EO 2 } aa 2g
EO 3
alcohol, 94%   50g
glycerine, 98%   20g

10 to 25 drops 3 times a day after meals.

While awaiting the results of the aromatogram, a preparation using those EOs rich in phenols (see page 84) may be used as a treatment of 'attack'. The EOs as determined by the aromatogram would then be used as part of a 'ground' treatment, which can last three or four (menstrual) cycles.

If essential oils are not tolerated well when taken orally, they can be mixed with hydrolisate of soya, or absorbed through a micro-enema (one which uses 100cc or less of liquid) (see Appendix 2). The schedule of doses can be adapted to the situation of the woman (for example, a woman who doesn't go home at noon, etc.). The first two preparations can also be individualized by replacing certain herbs with others selected according to their 'profile' or through the use of a *pendulum*. We should stress here that the use of a pendulum is not a matter of magic, but the intuitive use of one's stored herbal knowledge. Intuition can be drawn upon by emptying one's mind, asking a 'yes' or 'no' question, and allowing movement to come to the pendulum, which will indicate positive or negative. It works! (See References, *Guide de radiesthésie* and *La radiesthésie ou le pouvoir du pendule*.)

Let's look at the herbs which have not been discussed in earlier chapters:

Artichoke (*Cynara scolymus*)
Part used: leaves, not those usually eaten.
Properties: digestive, energizer and constructor, stimulant, hepatic tonic, cardiac tonic, blood depurative, anti-toxin, diuretic, suppresses breast milk production.

Indications: fatigue, over-work, growth, hepatic congestion and insufficiency, poisoning, intestinal infection.
Decoction: 1 fistful (30g) per litre liquid.

ATTENTION! *Don't throw away the cooking water of artichokes!* It is an excellent hepato-renal drainer (assuming the artichokes were not heavily treated – as are industrial artichokes), except for arthritics and women with gout and urinary infections.

Boldo (*Pneumus boldus*)
Part used: leaves.
Properties: aids secretion of bile, diuretic, general stimulant, hypnotic.
Indications: hepatic congestion and insufficiency, biliary lithiasis, urinary infection, hepatic insomnia.
Tincture: 20 to 100 drops each day before meals.

Fumitory (*Fumaria officinalis*)
Part used: entire plant.
Properties: tonic, depurative, hepatic drainer, softens arteries, anti-plethoric, vermifuge, aids formation of red blood cells. It is primarily a tonic and, in prolonged use, a depurative.
Indications: hepatic congestion, arteriosclerosis, plethora, arterial hypertension, intestinal parasites, dermatosis, gonorrhea.
Tonic: infusion: 50g per litre, 2–3 cups a day, 10 days per month (more than this will have the opposite effect).
Depurative: tincture: 20 drops before the two main meals.

Condurango (*Gonobolus condurango*)
Part used: bark of the stem, root.
Properties: aperitif, digestive, gastric analgesic.
Indications: lack of appetite, gastric afflictions, gastric pains of hepato-biliaries, considered by the ancients to be anti-syphilitic.

Turmeric (*Curcuma xanthorriza*)
Part used: rhizome.
Properties: friend of the gall bladder, anti-spasmodic, bactericide (especially for colibacilli, staphylococcus, streptococcus), and anti-convulsant.
Indications: hepatic insufficiency and congestion, biliary liathiasis and retention, hypercholesterolemia, intestinal fermentation, aerophagia, urinary infections, cellulite, difficult and painful periods, lactic insufficiency.
Infusion: 20g per litre, or in powder sprinkled into food.

Sweet briar (*Rosa canina*)
Part used: here fruit (rose hip), but also flowers and leaves.
Properties: tonic, astringent, hemostatic, diuretic, anti-anaemic, hormonal regulator.
Indications: diarrhoea, white vaginal discharge, haemorrhage, urinary lithiasis, avitaminosis, fatigue, spring cure, irregular cycles and other pituitary gland-ovarian dysfunctions.
In external use: (leaves and flowers): wounds, ulcers.
Tincture, or better still, bud glycerine macerate ID: 30 to 50 drops, mornings before eating.

Pansy (*Viola tricolor*)
Part used: flowers.
Properties: depurative, decongestant, diuretic, calms itching, tonic, anti-syphilitic (?).
Indications: diverse dermatoses (eczema, acne, psoriasis, dartre, boils . . .), phlebitis, haemorrhoids, herpes, hives, arteriosclerosis, nervous spasms.
Infusion: 50g per litre liquid, 2 to 3 cups a day.
Tincture: 10 to 25 drops before each meal.

And finally, even though it isn't a herb:

Clay rich in minerals and trace-elements, is a mineralizer, an equalizer, and an anti-toxic. Its use and powers are age-old knowledge. Clay is also an antiseptic, aids formation of scar tissues (vulnerary), and has a great power to absorb just about anything (colour, bad odour, toxins). Clay is very rich in silica and is therefore particularly indicated in all cases of demineralization and degeneration (fracture, tuberculosis, ageing, fatigue, cancerous 'ground', and anaemia).

Clay is used here in suppositories, but can also be applied in poultice (endometritis, benign tumours . . .) and taken orally. Clay for internal use must be finer and more carefully selected. In the evening, cover a teaspoon of clay with a glass of water. The next morning (the first 4 to 5 days only), drink the floating liquid. The other days, stir before drinking and drink all the water. Where use of clay leads to constipation, suspend use for two weeks (see also page 128).

∽ 7 ∾

Cervicitis and Ectropions

Cervicitis is an infection of the cervix, a fairly frequent gynaecological disease. One of the factors which may lead to these infections is the presence of an *ectropion*, or excrescence of the glands of the cervical canal which then push into the opening of the cervix. When this cervical tissue, which is adapted to a sterile environment, comes into contact with the vagina – which by definition is inhabited by germs – the result is a chronic inflammation. Viewed with the help of a speculum, the inflammation appears as a red ring around the opening of the cervix (see below).

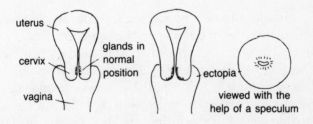

uterus
cervix
vagina
glands in normal position
ectopia
viewed with the help of a speculum

Ectropions are one reason for the cervix's lowered resistance to infections. Gonorrhea, too, is responsible for many cases of cervicitis (as are chlamydia, herpes and condylomas). Other factors include abortion, childbirth, the IUD and forgotten 'hygienic' tampons. A lowered resistance to infection may also be due to a lack of vitamins (how incredible that we can live in one of the world's richest countries and still lack vitamins! See Chapter 15).

❧

The signs

- A red and inflamed cervix which bleeds easily.
- Unusually abundant secretions which are thick and yellow-white, possibly with marked traces of blood;
- Possible back or lower abdomen pain, cramps, frequent and burning urination, painful periods.

Untreated, cervicitis may cause sterility, a pelvic infection (endometritis, adnexitis), a spontaneous abortion or difficulties in childbirth (dilation).

❧

What does modern western medicine propose?

An antibiotic is usually prescribed in order to eliminate the infection, but this treatment is one which can take several months. The antibiotic chosen depends on the germ involved (see under Vaginitis, page 65). For chronic cervicitis, acidic douches and surgery are proposed, as is cauterization (electro-coagulation, cryotherapy, micro-laser), and even conization (removing a small cone of the cervix), although this latter is controversial. There are those who are against it, and others who claim that it is a means of avoiding cancer of the cervix.

ॐ

What are the alternatives?

The first step is *disinfection* (see under Vaginitis), *which will take longer than for vaginitis*. The choice of herbs will depend on the germs involved. It is important that the disinfectant reach the cervix. For this reason, suppositories may be more effective than vaginal douches, which may be blocked by a fold in the vagina.

The next step is to encourage the formation of scar tissue (healing), through a daily application of lavender or rosemary honey. This honey must be of good quality and crystallized (hard). Vitamin E can also be used to paint the cervix (use Ephynal†, or take capsules intended for oral use and break them open).

Patience is another necessary element because the treatment of this kind of infection takes a long time. A series of treatments of several weeks each can be carried out over several months, with interruptions during menstrual bleeding.

Another preparation which can be used:

sweet almond oil	60g
wheat germ oil	20g
EO of thuya	4g
EO of cypress	4g

Soak a sterile tampon (not a Tampax, please! but a self-made tampon made of cotton wadding wrapped in a band of gauze, the end of which is left outside the vagina) in this liquid and place it against the cervix. Leave in place overnight.

Here we might mention:

Wheat (*Triticum vulgare*)
The whole grain (that is, unbolted) contains all the elements necessary to the proper functioning of our organism: calcium, magnesium, sodium, potassium, chlorine, iodine, arsenic, fatty phosphorus, starch (for warmth) and the vitamins A, B, E

(germ), K, D and PP, as well as the ferments necessary for digestion.

In addition, when sprouted, the quantity of these elements increases two to three times. Wheat is therefore an excellent food when there is a lack of vitamins, anaemia, growth and rickets, tuberculosis, pregnancy and breastfeeding, and the oil is a healing agent used locally.

In commercially available products, Weleda has a good preparation in its marjoram-balm suppositories of 1 or 3 grams, sold in series of 10.

For all pelvic complaints, cold water sitz-baths, taken in the morning and lasting several minutes, are very beneficial because they vigorously activate the circulation in this area.

If all these treatments fail, you should turn to a general treatment of the 'ground', and no longer concentrate solely on the cervix. (See also under precancerous states of the cervix, page 16).

৯ 8 ৯

Discharges and Itching
Outside Infection

The vagina is a constantly moist part of our bodies. The quantity of its secretions vary according to the phase of the menstrual cycle and the circumstances. The cells of the entire reproductive system leave the body through the vagina, as do menstrual blood and . . . babies!

After menstrual bleeding, the vagina is relatively dry. Secretions then become more abundant, liquid (creating a sensation of more lubrication), transparent, and stringy, resembling egg white, until ovulation. At this time a cervical mucus appears, secreted by the glands of the cervix. The function of the mucus is to provide an environment favourable to the survival of sperm and to help the sperm climb into the uterus. This mucus therefore marks the preovulatory and ovulatory stages. Observation of changes in this mucus allows us to pinpoint ovulation, either with the intention of preventing conception or, on the contrary, of favouring it. After ovulation, the secretions become white, opaque and are no longer stringy. The quality is variable, but the quantity tends to increase at the approach of menstrual bleeding. Apart from this general description, there is no norm for the quantity of discharge.

The abundance of discharge also varies according to diet. Dairy products, for example, increase it (as they increase bronchial secretions) and make it thicker. It is here that we become disagreeably aware of the eliminatory function of vaginal discharge!

113

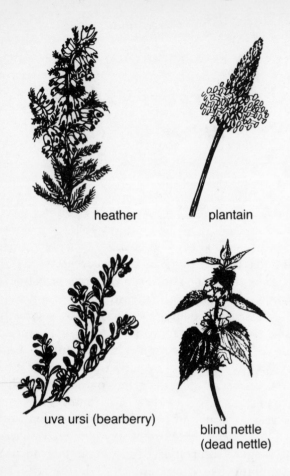

heather   plantain

uva ursi (bearberry)   blind nettle
                            (dead nettle)

Vaginal douches and obsessional hygiene also increase discharge (because they regularly destroy the lactic bacteria) and diminish defences. In addition, nylon underpants create a hot-house environment favourable to the growth of micro-organisms.

When the acidity (normally pH 4.5) changes, that is, when the discharge becomes more alkaline (the pH increases), the quality of the secretions changes and they may irritate the skin of the vulva, causing itching.

Since blood changes the pH of the vagina, there is often a recurrence of yeast and trichomonas infections after menstrual periods. The vaginal infection is not far off (see the figure on page 70).

At menopause, the vaginal secretions diminish. The mucus is less nourished by oestrogen; the vagina can even atrophy and itch. It should be noted, however, that sexual excitement also stimulates vaginal secretions and thus may offset lowered oestrogen.

After childbirth, too, there is an abrupt fall of oestrogen levels, and the signs may be temporarily similar. Depending on the woman, this transition may last weeks or even months, a fact which may not be graciously accepted by their partners.

For modern western medicine, these complaints do not exist or are not worthy of any preoccupation where an infection is not present – as if abundant discharge can't be a preoccupation in itself. Doctors therefore propose disinfectants or, at the very most, a lubricant if they think the problem is difficult penetration! During menopause and post-partum, they may propose a cream which contains synthetic oestrogens.

But let's turn to the herbs which can be useful here.

To begin with, there are the genito-urinary drainers, of which the first is preferably to be eaten raw:

Horseradish (*Cochlearia armorica*)
Part used: root.
Properties: appetite stimulant, aids secretion of bile, purgative, expectorant, anti-spasmodic, diuretic.
Indications: anaemia, deficiencies, lack of appetite, asthma, chronic bronchitis, white vaginal discharge.

To be eaten grated in salads or as an aperitif.

Heather (*Erica cinerea*)
Part used: flower tops.
Properties: diuretic and urinary antiseptic, depurative, sedative of urinary passages, astringent, anti-rheumatic.
Indications: cystitis, pyelonephritis, rheumatism, white vaginal discharge.
Decoction: 1 fistful per litre of water.

Tincture: 20 to 50 drops, once or twice a day.

Juniper (*Juniperus communis*)
Part used: berries, wood, leaves and essential oil of buds.
Properties: nerve tonic, digestive and excitant (berries), anti-septic, depurative, diuretic, anti-rheumatic, anti-diabetic, emmenagogue.
Indications: fatigue, infections of the urinary passages, gonor-rhea, intestinal fermentation, diabetes, painful periods, white vaginal discharge.
Buds: 20 to 30g per litre or 1 teaspoon per cup.
Tincture: 15 drops, 3 times a day.
EO: 0.1 to 0.2g per day.

Plantain (*Plantago*)
Part used: entire plant.
Properties: Purifier of blood, lungs and stomach, astringent, anti-inflammatory, increases coagulability of the blood. *In external use*: aids formation of scar tissue, decongestant, disinfectant.
Indications: weakness, weight loss, late development, haemor-rhage, haemophilia, bronchitis, pharyngitis, laryngitis, diar-rhoea, white vaginal discharge, nephritis*(?).
In external use: conjunctivitis, gingivitis, acne, wounds, crusty dermatoses, uterine inflammation, insect bites, snake bites, otitis.

Plantago is used in homoeopathy in dental neuralgia and night urinary incontinence. Used as a mouthwash, plantain creates a repugnance to tobacco.

Blind nettle (*Lamium album*)
Part used: leaves, flowers.
Properties: astringent, tonic specific to the uterus, vaso-constrictor, febrifuge, anti-inflammatory, depurative.
Indications: diarrhoea, bleeding between periods, white vaginal discharge, painful periods, haemorrhoids, varicose veins, cystitis.

Infusion: 1 teaspoon per cup.
Alcohol distillation: 2 to 4 teaspoons per day.
Decoction: 1 fistful per litre for use in vaginal douches.

Uva ursi (*Arbutus uva ursi*)
Part used: leaves, berries.
Properties: diuretic, antiseptic, acts against the oozing of pus, sedative of urinary passages, astringent.
Indications: inflammation of urinary passages, incontinence and retention of urine, diarrhoea, hematuria (blood in urine), white vaginal discharge.
Infusion: 1 fistful per litre.
Tincture: 10 to 15 drops per day.

Loosestrife (*Lythrum salicaria*)
Part used: flower tops.
Properties: astringent, anti-diarrhoea, hemostatic, antiseptic.
Indications: enteritis, bleeding between periods. *In external use*: uterine inflammation, white vaginal discharge, vulvar itching, leg ulcer, eczema.
Infusion: In internal use: 1 fistful per litre. *In external use*: 2 fistfuls per litre.

The herbs which we have already seen in preceding chapters and which are important here are: sage, blackcurrant, camomile, goldenseal, parsley, and lady's mantle.

And the groups of reserves (when none of the above works): sticklewort (*Agrimonia eupatoria*), St John's wort (*Hypericum perforatum*), English oak (*Quercus robur*), bramble (*rubus fructicosus*), and other herbs which we will discuss in future chapters.

Two cream-form preparations which may be useful:

tincture dwarf nettle	10g
tincture calendula	10g
cold cream	100g
hydrophile unguent	100g
castor oil	5g
EO niaouli	1g

EO cypress	1g
oil of camomile coctum	2.5g
EO lemon	1g

In certain cases, the use of lactic bacteria in other forms is enough.

Finally, clay may also be used, 4 tablespoons per litre, as a vaginal douche.

In cases of simple itching, the contraction and relaxation of the perineal muscles (anus, vagina, urethra) may also be useful, as are cold-sitz baths.

ॐ 9 ॐ

Bartholin Cysts and
Bartholinitis

When a shiny swelling of the lower half or third of the labia occurs, it is generally the result of an obstruction of the channel leaving the Bartholin glands. These two 1–2mm long glands are situated on each side of the vagina between the labia minor (inner lips) and the vaginal wall. Their purpose is to lubricate the entry of the vagina with their secretions.

The majority of occlusions (obstructions) are due to infections and subsequent abscesses. The inflammation takes care of itself, but where the Bartholin channel is damaged, causing a retention of secretions, a cyst is created.

The signs are pain and swelling, the degree of which depends on whether there is an infection, and on the degree of occlusion.

Examination: A culture will identify the germ involved, where infection is present.

It is important to distinguish between an abscess, a cyst, or, even more rarely, a cancer of the gland or of the canaliculus (primary or secondary to a vulvo-vaginal tumour).

⤳

What does modern western medicine propose?

Antibiotics, analgesics (such as aspirin), with plenty of rest. Surgery: excision and draining of the abscess. If the channels are chronically blocked, surgeons will create a pocket for the flow of the secretions of the gland. As a last resort, they will remove the gland. The prognosis is almost always good, they say.

⤳

What are the alternatives?

To begin with, clay as a local application, and rest. Clay has numerous properties. It is rich in minerals and trace elements, is a remineralizer, re-equalizer, anti-toxic, antiseptic, helps healing and is absorbant. It is used here externally. Clay is prepared in a glass, wood or porcelain dish (not metal or plastic). Cover the clay with water and wait until it is homogeneous. If you are in a hurry, clay can be mixed with a wooden spoon. Cold clay is applied directly to the skin and should be of such thickness that it dries in about an hour. A fresh poultice is applied two or three times a day in the beginning, then once a day. Clay is simply removed with water. If the skin becomes overly dry, a little oil can be added to the preparation or applied to the skin afterwards.

CAUTION: *Clay may aggravate the pain before relieving it; it is a true drainer*!

Clay may also be taken orally, in a preparation such as:

EO camomile		
EO thyme	(or according	
EO mint	to the	aa 1.5gg
EO lavender	aromatogram)	

tincture comfrey
tincture calendula } aa 10g
tincture witch hazel
green clay 5g
emulsion of sweet qsp 300g
   almond oil

In compresses, 2–3 times a day.

These treatments often make the excision of the gland unnecessary.

We have already seen the majority of these herbs in preceding chapters. Exceptions are: mint (*Mentha piperata*), here as antiseptic and antalgic, and thyme, preferably thuyanol-4 (*Thymus vulgaris*), also as antiseptic, vulnerary and revulsive (which drains secretions).

༃ 10 ༃

Endometritis and Salpingitis

Endometritis is an infection of the uterus. Its name derives from the endometrium, the mucous membrane which lines the interior of the uterine cavity and which is eliminated in each cycle. Salpingitis is a more serious infection involving the Fallopian tubes and the ovaries. It may even reach the envelope of the intestines, creating a danger of peritonitis. Clearly, in this chapter, we are dealing with serious infections. It is therefore recommended to avoid all amateurism and self-medication. This is a time to find an ally in healing!

Endometritis

Let's look first of all at endometritis.

This infection occurs most often after a vaginitis or cervicitis (for example, gonorrhea), the placing of an IUD, an abortion or childbirth, or after other intra-uterine interventions (such as hysterography).

The woman's temperature may be between 38° and 39°C (100.4° to 102.2° Fahrenheit), but fever may be absent.

Pain is situated above the pubis and is well centred; it may be preceded by a 'false cystitis' with frequent and burning urination. At palpation, pain may be accentuated at the release rather than upon pressure. Vaginal secretions are increased and resemble pus. Upon vaginal examination, the uterus and cervix are softened and *extremely* tender, and the adnexa are supple.

A conscientious health care worker can ask for the following complementary *tests*: a culture of the secretions with anti-biogram or aromatogram (see page 80), a blood sediment test (the rate at which sediment falls increase in relation to the number of white blood cells circulating in the blood), and a complete blood check-up.

Complications of endometritis pave the way for salpingitis (see below).

༄

What does modern western medicine propose?

In modern western medicine, treatment is a series of anti-biotics. For example, 3g of ampicillin per day (Penbritin†) or 750mg of amoxicillin 4 times a day, both for 10 days. Many other antibiotics may be used, but we'll stay with these two for now, as resistance to them has not yet developed. (Every antibiotic, after several years of general use, may lose its effect when there is a 'mutation' of the flora, which thus becomes resistant to that particular antibiotic.)

Particular attention must be paid to allergies to antibiotics and to previous use, including the brand name, of antibiotics. There is an absolute contra-indication in the case of a known allergy. Antibiotics increase fatigue. They can cause diarrhoea because they destroy intestinal flora. In this case, it is prefer-able to take the antibiotics during meals and not before, and to eat active yoghurt which reconstitutes the intestinal flora. However, we might mention here that certain recent research advises *against* the consumption of milk products during a tetracycline treatment; active yoghurts are perhaps not a panacea.

With antibiotic treatment, the pain ought to disappear by the 4th or 5th day, even at palpation.

ॐ

What are the alternatives

We do have alternatives. Below is the outline treatment that we at the women's health centre propose to women in good general health.

- *A lot of rest*, which means completely stopping work and bed rest;
- Diet: drink a lot of fluids and eat lightly. No cooked fats or animal proteins, increased vegetable proteins, guard against constipation by eating whole grains and bran.

     In the case of constipation, it is important to begin treatment with an enema.
- Local treatment: vaginal suppositories with the EOs indicated by the aromatogram.

EO x	
EO y	1 drop each
EO z	
tincture calendula	
tincture comfrey	0.03g
tincture goldenseal	
green clay	0.075g
excipient	qsp 1 suppository of 3g

Insert 1 suppository before going to bed.

Clay poultice on the lower abdomen, luke warm to cold, according to personal preference, for 3 to 4 days.

- General treatment: Cu or Cu-Au-Ag in trace element form: one dose per day, mornings before eating, then spaced out to three doses a week.

tincture sweet briar
tincture blackcurrant
tincture shave grass   } aa qsp 160ml
tincture pansy
tincture goldenseal

80 drops before each meal.

All these herbs have been discussed in preceding chapters. This treatment should be tried for 3 weeks. After that time the woman should be re-examined (see chronic infections, page 102).

Salpingitis

Let's turn now to acute salpingitis. This infection may follow endometritis or may develop as a result of the same circumstances which lead to endometritis.

In salpingitis, the two Fallopian tubes are attacked. They are congested or oedema is present. Pus-like secretions threaten to obstruct the tubes and create an abscess in the tubes or the ovaries.

Signs: temperature is between 39° and 40°C (102.2°– 104°F) with a lowered general state of health. The pain is intense and low, radiating into the thighs, anus and lower back. Vaginal secretions are not necessarily increased but frequently there is bleeding.

The abdomen is puffed out, 'breathes', and is sensitive in the supra-pubic zone to such a point that it may contract painfully and hinder a deep palpation. During the vaginal examination, the vaginal fornex are tender, as is the mobilization of the cervix. In particular, one or both tubes are swollen and tender. There may be a palpable mass indicating an abscess.

Tests: A culture, if there is a discharge. Except at the very beginning of the infection, the number of white blood cells is increased, averaging between 15,000 and 30,000 (the norm is less than 10,000). The rate of sedimentation is also increased.

Complications include an abscess of the Fallopian tubes, with the danger of a ruptured tube and a spreading of infection (parametritis and peritonitis), ovarian abscess, persistence of pain in the pelvis, persistence of swelling, painful periods, irregular periods and sterility. This last involves 20 per cent of women who have had salpingitis and is explained by the formation of adhesions and extensive scar tissue which alters the cells of the passage.

Other possible causes of these symptoms which must be considered (differential diagnosis) include: appendicitis, extra-uterine pregnancy, torsion (twisting) of a Fallopian tube, and spontaneous abortion.

When the pain is on the *right hand side* of the pelvis, it is difficult to distinguish between appendicitis and right salpingitis, and everyone makes a mistake occasionally. None the less, appendectomies are often abused, the number of these being, as is true of cesarians, directly proportional to the number of surgeons. This 'epidemic' is even more disquieting given that the appendix, like the tonsil, is a natural barrier against infection (they have the same cellular origin). There are certainly a number of acute cases where surgical intervention is indicated; fortunately, many others have a non-surgical solution. It all depends on the orientation, the financial and scientific ambitions, and the anxiety of the practitioner.

The decisive test is laparoscopy, which makes it possible to 'take a peek' into the pelvis. Under anaesthesia, a lighted hollow tube passes into the pelvis through an incision in the naval.

On the other hand, it is difficult to avoid antibiotics in acute salpingitis because its evolution is rather rapid and the fear of secondary sterility discourages slow treatment. In the case of gonorrhea, for example, it would be preferable to begin anti-biotics intravenously in order to accelerate recovery, something which involves brief hospitalization. In acute infections, certain western doctors also propose corticoids (derivatives of cortisone) in order to combat inflammation. Let us simply state that we do not agree with this practice.

Treatment outside of surgical cases:

- Rest should begin with 'complete bed rest' and last at least 4 weeks;
- Diet as for endometritis;
- Cu-Au-Ag in trace-element form, or Cu alone (see page 217);
- Antibiotics: 4g of ampicillin per day for three weeks and 600mg of Cleocin HCL† for ten days (to cover those germs which live without oxygen). In place of ampicillin, amoxicillin may be used; it has a better weight/result relation: 750mg four times a day for the same duration.
- The use of several essential oils (lemon, thyme, clove, lavender, mint, winter savory, niaouli, cinnamon, cajeput, hyssop) potentializes the effect of the antibiotics and counter-balances their side effects. As in cases of endometritis, the pain should cease by the 4th or 5th day and you can start spending progressively less time in bed at the end of a week or 10 days.

Chronic infections

Let's look now at the problem of chronic infections: an infection and local effects (including adhesions and fixed retroflexion) which reappear periodically. In chronic infections, the woman complains of episodic pelvic pain, pain upon penetration, painful periods, or of sterility. She has chronic discharge, the bladder is tender, and upon vaginal examination, a swelling which is generally bilateral can be detected.

In this situation, the repeated use of antibiotics will not improve things. It will in fact increase fatigue and diminish resistance.

This sparks anew an interest in *alternative treatments*:
- Rest is indispensable (although the difficulty of organizing

127

rest – depending on the social and family situation of each woman – needs to be recognized);
- Diet should be examined with an eye to relieving the digestive system and increasing immunity (see Chapter 15);
- Trace-elements: Cu-Au-Ag, alternating with Mg (magnesium);
- A local (suppositories of EO) and general treatment for endometritis;
- In addition, a hepato-renal drainer should be added such as:

tincture artichoke ⎫	
tincture boldo ⎬	aa 5g
tincture fumitory ⎭	
tincture condurango ⎫	aa 3g
tincture combretum ⎭	
tincture rosemary ⎫	aa 6g
tincture curry ⎭	
tincture shave grass	10g
tincture of olive tree (leaf) diluted at 10%	qsp 160ml

40 to 80 drops before the two main meals.

And a new herb:

Combretum (*Combretum raimbaultii*)
Part used: leaves.
Properties: helps the production of bile, diuretic, disinfectant, and purgative.
Indications: hepatic insufficiency, biliary lithiasis, and constipation.
Decoction: 10g per litre, 3 to 4 cups a day.
Fluid extract: 1 to 5g per day.

For another local application, clay poultices are very beneficial. Clay (see page 108) is used here as a local drainer, making use of clay's great capacity for absorption. Place the clay in a glass, wood or porcelain plate and cover with enough water to make a thick paste. If a spoon is used, it should not be either plastic or metal. Clay is applied directly to the skin. It can be covered with gauze or a towel. Drying time depends on the thickness of the applications which should range from ½ to 1cm. Once the clay is completely dry, it is rinsed off and thrown away. A poultice should be applied once a day for a minimum of 15 days per series. Clay can be lukewarm or cold depending on your personal preference.

In addition to their use in suppositories, essential oils (selected according to the aromatogram) can be taken orally or used in enemas. The EOs are mixed in 30cc of oil and inserted in the rectum (for the formula, see Appendix 2).

Against pain, a preparation such as the following may be used:

tincture oat	
tincture black horehound	} aa 6g
tincture valerian	
tincture hawthorn	
tincture peony	} aa 3g
tincture primrose	
alcohol distillation of balm qsp 120ml	

30 drops at a time (3 to 4 times a day) or 50 drops at night in case of insomnia.

Note that the valerian, like aluminium in trace element, acts here against anxiety and is not indicated in a hypo stage, like in melancholic depression; while passiflora and lithium in trace element acts as an anti-depressive and is not indicated in a hyper stage. The hyper-insomniac might be agitated by passiflora and lithium!

We have already discussed hawthorn and balm in the chapter on menopause, page 56, and peony in the chapter on irregular periods, page 42. Let's look at five other herbs.

Oat (*Avena sativa*)
Properties: oat is a reconstituting, energy- and tonus-giving grain which is well suited to cold countries.
Indications: It is recommended for children, convalescents and

those suffering from constipation. It has also been said to act in cases of sterility (?).

In tincture: oat is recommended for insomniacs. Although it may seem contradictory, oat in grain form is energizing, while the milk of oat, the straw infusion and the tincture are sedatives.

Black horehound (*Ballota foetida*)

Part used: flower tops.

Properties: anti-spasmodic, nervous re-equalizer, tonic.

Indications: anxiety, psychological problems stemming from menopause, sympathico-tonic states (certain insomnias, digestive spasms), whooping cough.

Tincture: 10 to 15 drops, two or three times a day.

Pasque flower (*Anemona pulsatilla*)

Part used: root, leaf, entire plant.

Properties: anti-spasmodic, special sedative action on the female genital organs.

Indications: nervous spasms, spasms of genital and gastro-intestinal organs, colds and spasmodic cough, painful periods, migraines.

Infusion: entire plant, 5g per litre, 2 to 3 cups a day.

Alcohol distillation: 20 to 50 drops a day.

CAUTION: *pasque flower when fresh is a poison*. When dry, it is innocuous.

Pulsatilla is one of the most widely studied homoeopathic remedies. The gynaecological indications of pasque flower are: periods which are delayed, scanty, or of thick black blood, amenorrhea after having had wet feet, painful periods, thick or yellow vaginal discharge, and ovaritis. It is indicated in particular in women with a tendency to tears, a need for consolation, and changing moods, who are timid, sweet, easy-going, and resigned.

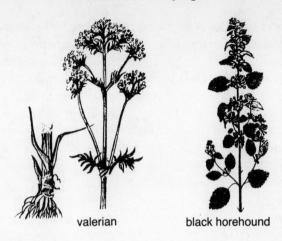

valerian   black horehound

Valerian (*Valeriana officinalis*)
Part used: root (entire plant).
Properties: re-equalizer of the nervous system, anti-spasmodic
 and anti-convulsant.
Indications: neurasthenia, hyperexcitability, infantile convul-
 sions, insomnia, hot flushes, asthma.
Tincture: 10 to 25 drops, 2 to 3 times a day.

CAUTION: *Valerian attracts and excites cats. Its exaggerated use
(in humans!) leads to addiction.*

Primrose (*Primula officinalis*)
Part used: root, entire plant, flowers.
Properties: anti-spasmodic, analgesic, expectorant, diuretic,
 vermifuge.
Indications: respiratory illness, headaches and migraines,
 neuralgia, dizziness, infantile convulsions, vomiting.
In external use: reabsorbs haematomas, even extensive ones.
Decoction of root: one teaspoon per cup of water.
Infusion: chopped plant and flowers in equal proportions.

As a final note, we will touch upon three methods useful in
treating the results of acute or chronic infections and to avoid
recurrences.

- *Short waves* (the only method recognized by modern western medicine) to avoid poor scar formation and adhesions.
- An *unblocking of the sacroiliac* (junction of the back and pelvis), if it is blocked. The sacroiliac may be unjammed by a passive mobilization or by manipulation which re-establishes a normal circulation of energy. For this treatment, go to a chiropractor or osteopath.
- *Acupuncture treatment of 'ground'.*

ॐ 11 ॐ

Cystitis

In general, urine and the urinary passages are sterile. Urinary infections and inflammation of the bladder are illnesses which attack primarily women because our anatomy (in this particular instance, it's true!) makes us more vulnerable in this respect. The channel between the bladder and the meatus (external orifice) is much shorter in women than it is in men. Thus the bladder is more easily contaminated by germs coming from the anus or vagina. For this reason, it is important to wipe from front to back after using the toilet, and not the reverse. Sexual relations with penetration are also a factor in cystitis, again by transporting germs – especially where anal penetration is followed by vaginal penetration without cleaning the penis or fingers in between. It is recommended to empty the bladder before and after sexual relations.

Apart from this, the best prevention is to drink a lot of fluids. This prevents statis, a factor favouring infection.

The bladder, like all organs, is a part of the whole organism. It is affected in particular by the nervous centres (vago-sympathetic, conscious and unconscious) and the upper urinary passages (kidneys and ureter), and by neighbouring organs (intestines, colon, uterus, and ovaries). Thus, the bladder may be the bearer of other health problems; an endometritis, for example, may begin with urinary signs, creating a false cystitis.

These elements explain the importance of such preliminary questions as: how long the signs have been present and under what circumstances they appeared; the date of the last menstrual period, the rhythm of the cycle and accompanying signs; and a medical history including operations (appendectomy), interventions of an obstetric (forceps delivery) or gynaecological (abortion, fibroids) nature, and previous medication (which antibiotics and in what quantity).

The signs of cystitis are well known: frequent and burning urination, pain above the pubis, especially after urination, and false need (three drops each time). Certain signs may lead one to suspect a pelvic infection: pain in the renal capsule, fever, nausea and vomiting, and blood in the urine.

A diagnosis of urinary infection is made only when a significant number of bacteria have been isolated in a culture. The clinical signs are less significant than this culture because there are forms of cystitis without symptoms and urinary signs without cystitis!

Most cases of cystitis are caused by a single germ. It can be assumed, therefore, when several germs grow in a culture, that there was a *contamination* of the culture by germs of the skin or elsewhere.

Tests: we talk about a 'urinary infection' when there are more than 100,000 colonies of the same species which grow in a culture. The easiest method for collecting a little urine without contaminating it is to urinate a first stream into the toilet, then to stop the flow (ouch! the cystitis!), releasing a second stream into a sterile container, finally finishing into the toilet.

In measuring the sediment (analysing the deposit of cells which precipitate to the bottom of the tube when the urine has been spun in a centrifuge for 5 minutes at 50,000 rotations per minute), we talk about 'cystitis' when there are more than 10 white blood cells per field when seen through the microscope.

The analysis of urinary pH (measure of acidity) is also indicative. We will come back to this point later.

What are the **dangers** of cystitis? The infection may recur and in particular may evolve into a pelvic infection (pyelonephritis or nephritis). Which women are particularly subject to cystitis? Pregnant women, women on the Pill, diabetics and all women whose immunity is low, and women with calculus or other obstruction (tumour).

The germs which we most frequently run into are: escherichia coli (the grand champion), proteus, klebsiellas, enterococcus, enterobacteria and pseudomonas.

$$\backsim$$

What does modern western medicine propose?

In modern western medicine, the treatment is essentially antibiotics, urinary disinfectants, or sometimes anti-inflammatories. Nowadays single-dose treatments are sometimes proposed, contrary to an earlier belief that a good antibiotic treatment had to be sustained for a minimum of 8 to 10 days in order to be effective. The antibiotics used are amoxycillin, 3mg; kanamycine, 500mg in intramuscular injection; or even sulphonamides (sulfisoxyzole, bactrim).

Single-dose antibiotics, a method which is both economical and less of a stress on the organism, supposedly relieves 50 per cent of all women. (For the others, the guilty germ must be isolated.) This method presents the same disadvantage as all 'blind' antibiotherapies: if it does not kill the germ responsible, it does it a favour by getting rid of its natural enemies and lowering the woman's immunological defences.

If an antibiotic must be used, it might as well be done knowing which one is the most effective, given that today's techniques of cultures and anti-biograms make this possible.

In the present of 10^3 to 10^4 germs (example: chlamydia), doctors propose doxycycline (Vibramycin†).

Finally, for modern western medicine, the only cause of the reappearance of infection is recontamination. Little, if anything, is said about the reasons for chronic illness. Those doctors who are more open, however, do recognize that it is the 'chronic' use of antibiotics which is at the root of numerous chronic illnesses.

჻

What more is there to understand?

The first step is to understand the mechanism of acidity. *The acid/base balance* is one of the key factors in the equilibrium of the organism (of its reactions and secretions).

Blood pH is situated between 7.32 and 7.43. Below this it becomes more and more acid; above, more and more alkaline (or basic). Urine has a pH between 7 and 7.5, like blood, as of the second urination of the morning. During the night it can drop to 5 or lower, the kidneys thus ridding themselves of their acidic waste. The important thing is for the blood pH to remain stable; this is done through breathing (elimination of CO_2) and the urinary system (elimination of excess acidity).

When a person stays in a closed space for several hours, her urinary pH drops to 5, while in open air it climbs to 7. Poor respiration causes an acidic urinary pH through an inadequate elimination of CO_2. If the intake of base-generation foods (see below) is insufficient and life too sedentary, the pH is permanently at 5 or below. This translates, before a full-blown illness, into fatigue, drops in energy level, headaches and a travelling ('rheumatic') pain . . . symptoms which are relieved simply by eating a more appropriate amount of base-generating foods.

Briefly, foods which are *acid generators* include: meat, white flour, sugar, tea, coffee, cacao, fats and egg white. *Base generators*, on the other hand, include fruits, vegetables, potatoes, milk, almonds, whole grain flours, and egg yolks. For further information, refer to the work of Dr Jackson, listed in the References, as well as Chapter 15).

In the majority of cases of cystitis (9 out of 10), the pH is too alkaline, that is, more than 7.5. However, don't jump to the conclusion that in cystitis the woman's diet is too alkaline. According to Dr Kousmine, excessive blood acidity may indicate over-alkaline urine. This may appear contradictory. However, marked alkalinity may in fact be the body's attempt, through alkaline salts, to compensate for not being able to eliminate acids through normal channels. For this reason, the situation is aggravated by the addition of acid.

How do we get the pH to return to normal? Well, you could take a teaspoon of citrate salts in a little water, 1 to 2 times a day, or a teaspoon of bicarbonate of soda in a little water, every other hour the first day and less often thereafter. This treatment should not exceed 3 days.

There is also a form of cystitis, called uric cystitis, where the urine is too acid. In this case, Vichy mineral water (carbonized mineral water with a high sodium bicarbonate content), leek juice or lemon juice help relieve symptoms.

In cystitis, the following foods should therefore be avoided: meat, shell fish, anchovies, sardines, preserves, sorrel, tea, coffee, sugar in any form, prunes, lettuce, carrots, green beans and spinach. On the other hand, *turnips* are valuable for their diuretic effect and ability to dissolve calculus and vitalize, *barley* as anti-inflammatory of urinary passages, and *leeks*, rich in alkaline salts, as an antiseptic, uric diuretic and laxative.

ꝶ

Let's come back to the now familiar world of herbs

Those which are the most helpful to us in this chapter are:

- those herbs which are anti-infectious and anti-inflammatory;
- those which are 'ground' herbs, drainers and diuretics; and
- those which are sedatives and tranquillizers.

(a) *Anti-infection*
In the foreground are *essential oils*, which are selected according to the aromatogram from among: rosemary, thyme, sage, winter savory, marjoram, oregano, hyssop, basil, lavender, fennel, cumin, coriander, cajeput, niaouli, pine,

eucalyptus (coli-bacillosis), *juniper* (except in a renal attack), clove, cypress, and cinnamon (used alone) . . . and *tinctures*: bilberry, heather, uva ursi, knot grass, feverfew, honeysuckle and poplar.

(b) *Anti-inflammatories*
Notable among these are papaya (*Carica papaza*), pineapple, saponaria, pellitory, and juniper.

(c) *Ground remedies*
Drainers and diuretics: shave grass, Mg, Cu, and other trace-elements, depending on the diathesis (see Appendix 3) clay (orally), honey and pollen. *Tincture*: goldenrod, birch, meadow-sweet, mouse-ear, couch-grass, linden (wood bark).

And drainers in poultice form: *clay* (see page 128) twice a day on the lower abdomen, unless it is unpleasant, or *cabbage* (4 thicknesses of leaves crushed with a rolling pin), twice a day for 2 to 3 hours.

(d) *Sedatives and tranquillizers*
In particular, willow and pasque-flower (urinary sedatives), but also oat, black horehound, passion flower, angelica, lavender, balm, primrose, valerian, hawthorn and peony.

༜

What can we propose as a treatment outline?

1. tincture bilberry
    tincture goldenrod   }   aa qsp 125ml
    tincture shave grass

40 drops 5 times per day the first 2 days, then 3 times a day.

EO lavender
EO oregano   }   or according to
EO clove   aromatogram   1g
94% alcohol   50g

98% glycerine   20g

30 drops after each meal. (See also page 84.)

2.   Crowberry (*Vaccinium vitis idaea*) bud glycerine macerate ID
     50 to 75 drops 3 times a day when acute,
     one a day when chronic.

     tincture mouse-ear:

     50 drops   5 times a day the first 2 days then
     3 times a day when acute,
     once a day when chronic.

     as a urinary sedative:
     alcohol distillation of willow   ⎫
     tincture pasque flower   ⎬   aa 10g
     alcohol distillation of balm   ⎭   qsp 60ml

     20 drops, 3 times a day.

There is also a homoeopathic remedy which is particularly
useful in cystitis: *cantharis* 4 CH, which may be taken:

* *either* by dissolving several grains in a glass of water, stirring
  with a plastic or wooden spoon and drinking a spoonful
  every half-hour, spacing out as soon as there is
  improvement;
* *or* 2 grains 4 times a day under the tongue.

For cystitis set off by a cold, aconite is especially well suited
as a treatment. To be taken in the same manner as cantharis.
It is of course more interesting to give an individualized
remedy in homoeopathy.
   Here are the details of a few herbs.

These are very closely related species.

Bilberry (*Vaccinium myrtillus*) and Crowberry (*Vaccinium
vitis idaea*)
Part used: leaves.
Properties: anti-diabetic, uric drainer, particularly powerful

anti-colibacillus action, favours circulation, regularizes digestion.

Indications: diabetes, excess urea, cystitis (especially caused by coli), circulatory problems, diarrhoea, constipation.

In all forms: fruit juice, *decoction*: 40g per litre, or *tincture and bud*: 50 to 75 drops, 3 times a day.

Mouse-ear (*Hieracium pilosella*)
Part used: entire fresh plant.
Properties: diuretic (eliminates urea and chlorides), stimulant, lowers cholesterol.
Indications: in cases of decrease of the quantity of urine in a fever, cardiac oedemas, excess urea, arteriosclerosis, fatigue (for example, convalescents).
Infusion: 100g per litre.
Tincture: 50 drops, 3 times a day.

Goldenrod (*Solidago virgaurea*)
Part used: flowers, entire plant.
Properties: hepatic and renal drainer, facilitates elimination of toxins, antiseptic, diuretic, sedative of urinary passages.
Indications: excess urea and cholesterol, urinary infection, uric liathiasis, albuminuria, hepatism, enterocolitis, eczemas.
Decoction: 1 fistful per litre, to be drunk in 1 or 2 days.
Tincture: 25 to 60 drops, 3 times a day.

In homoeopathy, *solidago* is a hepato-renal drainer – a remedy particularly indicated when there is a painful tenderness upon pressing the two costo-lumbar angles.

White birch (*Betula alba*)
Part used: leaves, bark, sap.
Properties: diuretic (eliminates chlorides, urea, uric acid), depurative, digestive, brings down a fever.
Indications: cardio-renal oedemas, hyperozotemia, hypercholesterolemia, rheumatism or excess uric acid,

nephretic lithiasis and colitis, obesity, arthritis, arterial hypertension, intestinal parasites, arteriosclerosis.
Tincture: 10 to 40 drops, 2 to 3 times a day.

One can use the *betula pubescens* in glycerin macerate of buds ID 30 to 50 drops a day, for relieving breast tension.

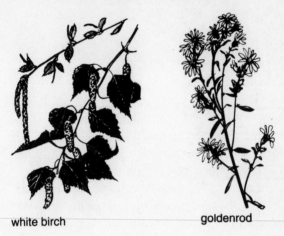

white birch   goldenrod

᧵ 12 ᧵

Endometriosis

Endometriosis is a gynaeco-
logical ailment whose cause is unknown to modern western
medicine and which involves the growth of endometrial tissue
(tissue lining the uterus) outside the uterine cavity. As in the
uterus, these tissues follow the menstrual rhythm, proliferating during the cycle and bleeding during periods – thus
provoking a serious local inflammation. Endometriosis occurs
in women of child-bearing age and generally in women who
are *hyperfolliculinemic* (see page 12).

Although endometriosis is hormone-dependent, it is inhib-
ited by pregnancy. As we understand it today, endometriosis is
sustained by the ovarian hormones, but not necessarily acti-
vated by them. We might add that endometriosis is aggravated
by the use of IUDs.

In 80 per cent of cases, these abnormal tissues are found on
the Fallopian tubes and the ovaries; in 40 per cent of cases, on
the uterine wall. Other possible sites are: the recto-vaginal
dividing wall, the pelvic peritoneum, the vaginal fornix, the
bladder, the cervix and, in rare cases, the lungs. This clearly
demonstrates that the disease spreads not only locally, but is
transported by the lymph nodes or the blood.

The sign of endometriosis is severe pain during menstrual
bleeding which radiates into the thighs and sacrum, and which
is calmed neither by rest nor by the usual analgesics. Periods
are longer and more abundant, even to the point of haemorrhaging. In cases of implantations in the digestive system,

there may be bleeding from the rectum. Sterility is frequent. The bladder is tender and urination painful. The urine is clear.

Tests: Pelvic examination will reveal a uterus which is tender, ovaries increased in volume and painful, and a painful swelling in the recto-vaginal wall. With the help of a speculum, bluish clusters can be seen, especially at the end of the cycle. Otherwise, exploratory laparoscopy (possibly cytoscopy or rectoscopy) will make diagnosis possible.

⤳

What does modern western medicine propose?

The treatment of modern western medicine aims at suppressing the work of the ovaries through hormone therapy. There are differing schools of thought: some doctors prescribe combined oral contraceptives, others progestogens. In both cases, bleeding due to interruptions in taking the Pill is suppressed. *Danazol* (Danocrine†, Danol† in UK) is another favourite because it has neither oestrogen nor progesterone activity which might sustain the disease. It is, rather, an inhibitor of all pituitary gland hormones. The ovaries thus do not receive the order to secrete oestrogens and progesterone, and periods are suppressed. This treatment is not innocuous, however, because it produces certain androgenic side-effects: hot flushes, acne, body hair, and possibly an irreversible modification of the voice. In addition, because it also inhibits secretion of the anti-diuretic hormones of the pituitary gland, it is contra-indicated for those suffering from cardiac or renal diseases.

Pregnancy would produce the best hormonal effect, but it can't really be called a treatment!

Along with analgesics, psychotherapy and possibly surgery might be recommended. There are diverse approaches in surgery as well, although all attempt to be more or less conservative in terms of what is removed. In the majority of cases, the uterus and the Fallopian tubes are removed. Depending on the extent of the invasion, the ovaries or a part of them may be spared. Other surgeons believe that the ovaries can be the point of departure for a new endometriosis, however, and prefer to remove them completely, causing premature menopause. The removal of parts of the digestive system may also be considered necessary, depending on the individual case.

ॐ

What are the alternatives?

We followed several women at the women's health centre suffering from endometriosis, so far with good success. The infection seems to be more frequent in the United States, where it attacks 3 to 15 per cent of the women of child-bearing age (*Ob. Gen. News*, October 1980).

Dr Catherine Kousmine, on the other hand, has had many years of experience with this disease, and maintains that its correction is possible through changes in diet and vitamin therapy. It is in any case always necessary to begin treatment by consideration of these aspects. (Speaking of diets, we might again raise the question of whether the exaggerated use of hormones in raising calves, chickens, and the like is not partly responsible for these hyperfolliculinemic (hyperoestrogenemic) diseases.)

Herbs and trace-elements may also produce vital support.

Treatment has several objectives:

- to brake* hyperfolliculinemia with:
  tincture: gromwell, lady's mantle, chaste tree, yarrow, blackcurrant.
  EO: cypress, hyssop, angelica, oregano, geranium.
  Placental extract, like Placenta ICH in organotherapy, may also be effective.

- to calm the pain:
  tincture: sweet clover, willow, black horehound, hawthorn, primrose, comfrey, raspberry, yellow melilot, goldenseal, witch hazel, gelsemium.
  EO: tarragon, basil, angelica, lavender, rosemary, camomile.
- to treat the 'ground':
  trace-elements: Mg (magnesium), Li (lithium), Zn (zinc), Cu (copper), Mn (manganese).
  Tincture: blackcurrant, shave grass, raspberry, bramble, wild pansy.
  Local applications of clay are helpful.

Let's look at some of these herbs more closely, beginning with two which are progesterone-like, having already discussed oestrogen-like herbs in the chapters on periods and the menstrual cycle (Chapters 1 to 5).

Gromwell (*Lithospermum officinalis*)
Part used: entire plant, seeds.
Properties: diuretic, dissolves calculus (?), inhibitor of pituitary gland, progesterone-like.
Indications: urinary and biliary lithiasis, rheumatism, gout, amenhorrhea and all situations in which one wants to imitate* a cycle, endometriosis. *In external use*: foreign bodies in the eye.
Infusion: 2 tablespoons per cup, 3 cups a day.

Chaste tree (*Vitex agnus castus*)
Part used: leaves.
Properties: anti-spasmodic, vago-sympathic equalizer, general and genital sedative, progesteron-like.
Indications: palpitations, pain in the solar plexus, dizziness, intestinal spasms, insomnia, 'psychological malaise expressed by a gynaecological ailment' (Leclerc), amenorrhea and all situations in which one wants to imitate* a cycle.

White willow (*Salix alba*)

Part used: male flowers, leaves, bark.

Properties: genital sedative, anti-neuralgic, anti-spasmodic, calmative, febrifuge, digestive tonic.

Indications: painful periods, nervousness, anguish, biliary lithiasis, gastric hyperacidity, fever.

Infusion of male flowers (catkin) or leaves: 1 teaspoon per cup, 1 to 3 cups a day.

Decoction of bark: 20 to 35g per litre, 2 to 3 cups a day.

Most of the other herbs have already been described in earlier chapters.

An example of a possible treatment outline and its results:

- Mn-Cu (trace-elements chosen according to diathesis; see Appendix 3);
- placental extract (Placenta ICH, as a drink or in suppository form), every other day;
- during the first phase of the cycle: tincture of blackcurrant, raspberry, shave grass, bramble, wild pansy (in equal amounts, 40 drops twice a day);
- during the second phase of the cycle: tincture of gromwell, lady's mantle, yarrow, chaste tree, goldenseal (in equal quantities, 80 drops twice a day);
- during menstrual bleeding:

tincture piscidia	
tincture gelsemium	aa 3g
tincture pareira brava	
tincture witch hazel	
tincture comfrey	aa IO
tincture primrose	

tincture of raspberry diluted at 10% qsp 100ml
100 drops 3 times a day.

In a case treated by a women's health centre, the first period under this treatment lasted seven days. It was painful but lasted less time than previous periods. The second period lasted four days. It was less painful and then only for a few hours. The third period was a little painful during the night, but did not need any medication. Since the fourth period under this treatment, the woman has had no pain whatsoever and has taken no medication, including herbs.

The treatment was none the less maintained for an additional four months with a change of trace-elements. The woman made important changes in her diet and there was a dialogue during these months which cannot be retransmitted here.

In case you're having doubts about whether it was really endometriosis, we will point out that the diagnosis was made by the Polyclinic of Gynecology of the University of Geneva, based on laparoscopic examination. The woman concerned had already tried all the hormonal treatments, and had found she could not tolerate them due to circulatory problems.

Since ending this treatment, she just takes tincture of raspberry from time to time, and is in perfect health!

If this is not enough, energetical acupuncture or homoeopathy can be of great help.

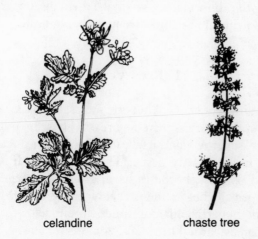

celandine   chaste tree

ॐ 13 ॐ

Benign Tumours

In this chapter I will try to describe the non-cancerous tumours appearing in women, including breast cysts, uterine fibromas, ovarian cysts and cervical dysplasias.

This chapter – with its descriptions of alternative treatments – is especially important because modern western medicine has no medical treatment for these diseases. It can only try surgery, removal of the tumour or the entire organ, electrocoagulation, or freezing. 'Treatment' is limited to destroying the abnormal cells to make them disappear.

The following are the most frequent benign tumours.

(1) Breast cysts

There are different kinds of hypertrophias, that is, an exaggerated development of tissue in the breast. These may attack the epithelial tissue, the gland itself, its galactophor ducts (which direct the milk) or fatty tissue. The breast, which is usually supple and painless, becomes hard, grainy and tender, even painful, especially before menstrual bleeding. As the development of the hypertrophia continues, an entire section of the breast becomes hard. These hard zones can be found in both breasts, although not necessarily in a symmetrical fashion. The first sign may also be a single and well-defined cyst.

Modern medicine does have one extraordinary thing to

offer: the possibility of knowing what kind of tumour is involved through mammography (X-ray negative of the breast) or thermographies (a colour chart depicting the temperature of the breast). This latter has the advantage of not irradiating the breasts, but without other tests both these techniques are less reliable. The most reliable method is the needle biopsy, as long as the puncture is done directly into the tumour itself. An analysis of the cells is indispensable for identifying the tumour.

Of course, surgeons love to say that one can be sure of a diagnosis only when the entire mass has been removed! They often suggest not waking women up between the removal of the cyst and the removal of the breast if the tumour turns out to be malignant. They say that it is to avoid a second anaesthetic, but perhaps they are scared silly that the intervention might cause a spread of cancerous cells through the blood or lymph glands. Every woman has the absolute right to know the diagnosis, and to have some time to think through her choice of treatment. Hopefully surgery is becoming more 'conservative' (removing as little as possible). It remains essential to prepare yourself well (both emotionally and physically) before an operation.

But let's stay with the possibility that the woman will have the pleasure of waking up with both breasts – and will perhaps forget the entire episode and the warning it represented.

A tendency to cysts triples the risk of cancer of the breasts! In addition, the hard masses make a proper breast examination difficult – which might mean a delay in detecting a cancerous growth. (For information on breast examination, see the next chapter.)

〜

What are the 'ground' considerations for cysts?

Generally, cysts form in women who absorb more than their body is able to metabolize and eliminate. The issue is not only one of quantity, but also of quality: a diet consisting of excessive animal proteins (meat, butter, milk, eggs, cheese) and foods which are over-refined (such as white flour and white sugar), over-cooked, and over-rich in butter and cream, is a diet lacking in minerals and vitamins and far too heavy. Women with a tendency to cysts also have a tendency to constipation and *difficult elimination* because of liver and kidney deficiencies, which are signalled by headaches, pimples, bloatedness, and increased discharge from the eyes, bronchial tubes and vagina.

Dr Catherine Kousmine has treated degenerative illnesses such as cancer, evolutive chronic polyarthritis and multiple sclerosis for over 40 years. According to her theory, when the *liver* is no longer able to disintoxicate the organism, a 'second liver' is created in the form of a cyst, fibroid, or articular inflammation where the toxins are stored. For this reason, we in naturopathy are not eager to remove cysts, as we would all other benign tumours, before changing this tendency. We consider the cyst to be performing a role in maintaining the organism's equilibrium.

Another point common to women with a tendency to cysts is a circulatory weakness. This can be manifested by heavy legs, varicose veins, or haemorrhoids. Where the circulation is poor, the cellular exchanges take place even more erratically, hence the appearance of an abnormal mass.

There are, however, two other key elements in the tendency to cysts: one is the *hormonal interplay*, the other is *stress*.

It is known that the breasts are influenced by sex hormones (FSH, LH, LTH, oestrogens, progesterone and prolactin). They may be swollen, for example, and more sensitive at the end of the menstrual cycle, when the level of hormones in the blood is at its highest (see Chapter 1). Thus, it is possible that the hormonal instructions to the mammary gland become chaotic due to a relative imbalance between the oestrogen and progesterone hormones (hyperoestrogenemia or hypoprogesteronemia).

Stress is certainly not the easiest element to improve without changing your way of life. It would appear that in cases of cysts, a state of nerves increases the permeability of the intestinal mucous membrane to toxins which, as the liver is unable to eliminate them, move into the breast.

Alternative treatment therefore aims at improving digestion, elimination and circulation. This increases the cellular exchanges and thus the rate at which the body 'cleanses' itself. The first stage – the fundamental one – is dietary change. The best diet is one which destroys the food as little as possible. This means raw fruit and vegetables, whole grains and cereals, and vegetable proteins rather than animal ones. Regular meals (when possible), with the larger meals in the morning and at noon rather than in the evening, especially at the end of the cycle, are also important. Locally, clay works wonders through its draining properties. Users should be warned, however, that the pain may get worse before it gets better. Clay is applied to the breasts in poultices of ½cm thickness and left to dry. Clay is mixed with water which is lukewarm or cold, depending on personal preference. Repeat once a day, except for the week of menstrual bleeding.

Among the valuable herbs in this chapter, let us cite:

- *for digestion*: tincture: burdock, senna, artichoke, borage, rhubarb, liquorice, elder, mallow, mint;
- *to improve liver function*: tincture of dandelion, garlic, boldo, condurango, turmeric, combretum, linden, rosemary;
- *to improve urinary function*: tincture of shave grass, mouse-ear, birch, linden wood-bark;
- *to improve circulation*: tincture of climbing ivy, service-tree, horse chestnut, cypress, cowped, bilberry, witch hazel (and the key herb in haemorrhoids, goldenseal);
- *hormonal regulators*: glycerine macerate of raspberry, blackcurrant, tincture of sweet briar;

- *tranquillizers (for lack of anything better)*: tincture of valerian, balm, horehound, oats, pasque flower, hawthorn, peony, primrose and passion flower.

ॐ

The following outlines one possible treatment

- a herb with a hormonal influence: raspberry (if periods are abundant), blackcurrant (if periods are scanty) or betula pubescens in glycerine macerate of bud ID, 50 drops each morning before eating.
- an association of herbs to aid elimination:

tincture artichoke	
tincture boldo	aa 5g
tincture fumitory	
tincture condurango	
tincture combretum	aa 3g
tincture rosemary	
tincture turmeric	aa 6g
tincture shave grass	10g
tincture of olive tree (leaf) diluted to 10%	qsp 160ml

40 drops before meals at noon and in the evening.

- an association of circulatory herbs, if this system is weak:

tincture bilberry	
tincture of cypress	aa 3g
tincture cowped	
tincture witch hazel	
tincture ragwort	aa 6g
tincture goldenseal	
tincture horse chestnut	
alcohol distillation service-tree	qsp 90ml

30 drops, 3 times a day.

- a tranquillizing combination, if the need arises (to be used for short periods of time only):

tincture oat	
tincture black horehound	aa 6g
tincture pasque flower	
tincture valerian	
tincture peony	
tincture hawthorn	aa 3g
tincture primrose	
alcohol distillation balm	qsp 120ml

50 drops before bedtime.

- locally, clay in series of 3 weeks (interrupting for week of menstruation). Massaging the upper part of the breasts to the thorax improves circulation.
- and finally, possibly a trace-element, depending on the diathesis.

Results: In our experience, this type of treatment has not caused a great number of cysts to shrink, but it has caused them to soften and to stop their evolution.

(2) Uterine fibroids

The fibroid of myoma is one of the most common uterine tumours. It is most often the muscle which is fibrosed, but the fibroid may also be constituted by one or several well-defined masses in another part of the uterus.

A fibroid is usually painless. Although the woman may feel its weight or the pressure that it causes when it is of considerable size, it is often not noticed when small. The first sign is very abundant periods – almost to the point of haemorrhaging. This is because the fibrosed uterine muscle loses its elasticity and is no longer able to contract as well. At this stage, fibroids are easily detected by bi-manual palpation (two fingers in the vagina and the other hand on the abdomen). The uterus is enlarged (it can reach as far as the navel) and much firmer than usual. A spherical mass may be palpable.

Treatment of women who consult doctors because of this bleeding is: a biopsy, to determine the nature of the tumour, and curettage (the removal of the mucous membrane lining the uterus), to bring an end to the bleeding. After two to three curettages, the gynaecologist will propose removing the uterus because he doesn't have any medical treatment to offer. Technically, the removal of the tumour alone is not always possible because the masses are often multiple and intertwined with the uterine muscle.

One type of tumour which can be seen during an examination with a speculum is the *polyp* which protrudes from the cervix. It is fragile and bleeds easily.

This type of tumour develops in women 25 to 45 years of age; it is linked to the production of sex hormones and more precisely to hyperfolliculinemia (hyperoestrogenemia), as is the exaggerated bleeding which often accompanies it.

✢

Why fibroids?

The mechanism at the origin of this kind of tumour is the same as that of the cyst found in the breast, that is, a 'second liver'. Now, why does the organism choose the uterus and not the breast? Well, that's a mystery! The schools of medicine which are more individually-based approaches, such as homoeopathy and acupuncture, are able to ask this kind of question. For us, it may be that in this case it is the pelvis which is the site of a *poor circulation of energy*. A low level of energy in the pelvis is accompanied by a tendency to gain weight in this area (cellulite) and by pelvic congestion at the end of the cycle. This phenomenon, common to so many women, emphasizes the extent to which this part of the body, which is also that of sex and sexuality, is ill-considered in our civilization. Apart from tackling the mountain of prejudices and taboos to change this, two simple methods may be proposed: one consists of putting one's buttocks in a pan of cold water every morning for two to three minutes. This 'gripping' method activates the local circulation in a very beneficial manner! The other method is the 'yoga' of Aviva Steiner (already discussed on page 29), the basic exercise of which – rocking the pelvis – encourages a normal circulation of energy. Breathing also plays an important role in these exercises: you are instructed to imagine that you inhale and exhale through your vagina!

The treatment for fibroids has the same goals as that for breast cysts:

- improve diet;
- brake the hyperfolliculinemia (hyperoestrogenemia);
- encourage the hepatic and renal elimination;
- improve general and local circulation;
- combat stress (if necessary).

Below is our treatment outline. This treatment is equally useful for polyps or polyposes which are to be considered as part of this chapter.

- to brake hyperfolliculinemia, a more complete preparation than that used in cases of breast cysts; between the following plants:

tincture blackcurrant	
tincture gromwell	
tincture lady's mantle	
tincture chaste tree	aa 10g
tincture yarrow	
tincture wild pansy	
tincture sequoia	
alcohol distillation thyme	qsp 120

One teaspoon each morning before eating;

- a drainer, as described on page 152;
- a circulatory preparation, such as is described on page 152;

- in cases of bleeding:

tincture comfrey	
tincture verbena	
tincture barberry	
tincture rhatany	aa 10g
tincture witch hazel	
tincture broom	
alcohol distillation anise	qsp 60ml

100 drops, 3 times a day;

- Mn (manganese) in trace-element form, 3 to 4 doses a week;
- local applications of clay, in series of 3 weeks alternated with 1 week of rest (the week of menstrual bleeding) (see page 108 for how to prepare clay);
- a tranquillizing preparation, if necessary.

Sequoia (*Sequoia gigantea*)
Yes, we are talking about the great Californian tree which can live 2,000 years and more! The sequoia is a tonic and clearly acts upon the uro-genital sphere. It is indicated in cases of fibroids in women (and hypertrophy of the prostate in men).

Bud glycerine macerate: 50 to 150 drops a day.

Results: This is without a doubt one of the most successful chapters on gynaecological phytotherapy because all the fibroids in women between 40 and 50 years of age which we have treated have improved within 6 months, even if a secondary treatment has sometimes had to be maintained for a year and a half.

(3) Ovarian cysts

These benign tumours are formed in the interior itself of ovarian tissue, forming a cavity filled with a more or less clear liquid. There are also dermatoid cysts, without liquid, made of tissue similar to that of teeth, hair, etc.

WARNING: *a Pill prescription whose dosage is too low, that is, a Pill which does not have enough of an inhibiting effect on the pituitary gland, may cause an ovarian cyst!*

Beyond this, it is not known why an obstruction occurs and a cyst is created in the ovary. Whether it be the result of the follicle-stimulating hormone's (FSH) influence, that is, during the first phase of the cycle, or under the influence of the luteinizing hormone (LH) during the second phase, it may be that one stage does not take place and that a cyst forms and regresses spontaneously. Such a cyst is called 'functional'.

A cyst may be detected during an annual examination, or be signalled by increased discharge, problems with bleeding or with the cycle (premenstrual signs), by pain in the pelvis, sterility, or even by peripheral circulatory problems.

The most common signs are severe pain, urinary retention, and discomfort and difficulty in having bowel movements. An enlarged ovary may be felt at palpation. An ovary may be transitionally enlarged without it being abnormal, but if the mass persists beyond two cycles, it can be considered to be a tumour.

In the case of an ovarian mass, the first step is to distinguish between an inflammatory lesion which is the result of a chronic infection (for example, gonococcic abcess), a benign tumour (liquid or functional cyst), dermoid or haemorrhaging cyst, an emergency situation (torsion of a cyst, extra-uterine pregnancy), salpingitis or endometriosis, or finally, a malignant tumour! As you can see, this list of possibilities is a bit long. Narrowing it down requires a specialist, who quite often will perform an exploratory laparoscopy or laparotomy (opening of the abdomen) in order to confirm a diagnosis. It should be noted here that non-surgical treatment is possible for functional cysts and benign tumours (ovarian, fibroids, and sclero-cystic dystrophy). Although it is true that functional cysts disappear spontaneously, this is no reason not to treat them!

At this point, I'd like to take a moment to object to the

all-too-frequent habit of modern western doctors of prescribing the Pill in order 'to give the ovaries a rest'. It is highly doubtful that this 'rest' facilitates the resumption of a normal cycle afterwards.

ॐ

But what can be done otherwise?

Yet again, herbal medicine can be useful, with the following:

- *'brakes'*: *tincture*: chaste tree, gromwell, yarrow, blackcurrant. *EO*: cypress, hyssop, angelica, oregano, sage, winter savory, geranium and, even though they are not herbs, mammary and placental extracts.
- *tranquillizers*: *tincture*: sweet clover, willow, black horehound, hawthorn, passion flower, pasque flower, valerian, celandine, peony, meadowsweet.
  EO: tarragon, neroli, oregano, basil, angelica, lavender.
- *antalgics*: *tincture*: primrose, gelsemium, goldenseal, witch hazel, comfrey, barberry, raspberry, tansy, yellow melilot.
  EO: rosemary, camomile, mint.
- *drainers*: tincture hepato-ball bladder: tincture black radish, boldo, and dandelion. *Urinary*: tincture ruscus, mouse-ear, shave grass, meadowsweet, goldenrod, poplar.

Trace-elements can also be useful: Mg (magnesium), Li (lithium), Mn-Cu (manganese-copper), Zn (zinc), Co (cobalt).

Finally, and complementarily, we mention clay again, in poultice and orally (see page 108 and under References).

We have had good results in chronic ovarian cysts with homoeopathy.

(4) Dysplasias of the cervix

These microscopic benign tumours of the cervix have a special place in this chapter: they exist only because the technique of the Pap smear exists. At benign stages, they do not cause any signs and a woman cannot be aware of them. A cervical smear can detect all changes in the cervix – such as dysplasias – some of which may become cancerous in the future. Dysplasias, therefore, fit under the category of benign tumours, which is why they appear in this chapter.

Most often, modern western doctors do not inform women of the abnormal cells in order not to frighten them, and propose:

- *for dysplasias* (light, moderate, marked): electrocoagulation, cryotherapy (freezing), or, most recently, laser rays;
- *for marked dysplasia*: the conization or removal of a cone of the cervix.

In this way, women may know that they have once had an electrocoagulation, but most often do not know if it was for a dysplasia or an ectropion! It should be mentioned that cryotherapy leaves a scar on the cervix which may interfere with Pap smear results. In addition, repeated cryotherapies can hinder natural dilation at childbirth.

From the moment when the stamp 'We haven't seen any suspected malignant cells' no longer appears on the results of the cytology lab, we at the women's health centre prefer to tell women the name of the cellular anomaly.

Zone of regeneration: Following an attack of the mucus of the cervix, there is a reconstruction of the mucus with normal cells.

Zone of junction: Intermediate zone between the glandular zone (endocervical) and non-glandular (exocervical), forming a white border which does not trap the iodine.

Cervical dysplasias

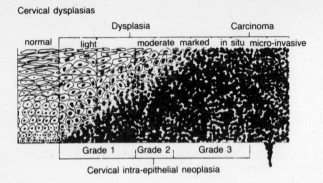

Ectropion: Overflow of the endocervical mucus on to the surface of the cervix (exocol). This mucus being fragile and less prepared to tolerate the irritations of the vaginal milieu, is often inflamed, even to the point of haemorrhaging. An ectropion may be due to a pregnancy, an abortion, or to oral contraceptives.

Leucoplakia: This whitish patch on a mucous membrane may have various origins. A layer of keratine is formed and comes off in patches or squamas.

Epidermal metaplasia: Transformation of the epithelium (layer covering the mucous membrane), normally not corneous, into an epithelium which resembles skin (dermatoid). This generally happens in response to a chronic irritation of the mucous membrane, and is a completely normal means of defence.

Parakeratosis: Change in the appearance of the epithelium which thins and forms more keratine (horny layer, cf. epidermal metaplasia). It is not considered pre-cancerous.

Accuminatum condylomas: Warts formed by a local proliferation of the mucous membrane. Of a viral origin, they can be found on the vulva, vagina, cervix, anus or penis.

Polyp of the cervix: Glandular proliferation developing in the cervix or in the uterus and protruding through the cervix. There is often an associated dermatoid metaplasia, and the surface of the polyp may ulcerate or bleed (bleeding upon contact). Malignant transformation very rare.

Dysplasia: Transformation of the cells in their form and organization, and increases in mitoses (increased proliferation, larger nuclei). Three stages can be distinguished according to the severity of the alteration: slight, moderate, or marked. Malignant transformation possible, but not certain. Spontaneous remission possible.

Our aim here is to demystify and de-dramatize this vocabulary, and put information at the disposal of the women themselves. Putting this attitude into practice is far from simple. Experience has taught us to be prudent and delicate in our explanations, without giving up our cherished principle of sharing information.

From the moment of diagnosis of slight dysplasia, while still offering the choice of the methods of modern western medicine, we propose the following alternatives:

We used to propose a preparation for local use: tampons soaked in the following solution and placed against the cervix during the night (formula for the solution already seen in cervicitis and ectropions, page 111).

sweet almond oil	60g
wheat germ oil	20g
EO thuja	10g
EO cypress	10g

However, after several months, we stopped using this preparation systematically because we observed that this daily practice, although very effective, caused women to be too conscious of their cervix. Despite this, one should mention the good results obtained on dysplasia related to plain lesion like condyloma with CTEO of niaouli (melaleuca quinquinervia), see page 92.

In general, we prefer to attend to problems such as diet and other risk factors of cancer (taking the Pill, cigarettes, other drugs, environment, etc.). As a preventive measure, a draining preparation can be used, the formula for which we have from Drs Tetau and Bergeret (see References). It can be effective, although it has the disadvantage of encouraging an attitude of passive consumption – counter-productive in this type of problem:

tincture mouse-ear	
tincture dandelion	aa 30g
tincture garlic	
tincture celandine	aa 20g
tincture buckthorne	

20 drops, 3 times a day.

Undeniably, what is most important is to investigate the 'ground' of the woman, her possible tendency to cancer, and her other strengths and weaknesses, and decide how to act at this level. Fortunately, the naturopathy world today has several techniques for approaching this problem. Among them: iridology (examination of the iris of the eye), the Heitan-Lagarde test, Vincent's bioelectric, sensitive crystallography (see References), and, finally, the Vernes tests, which I will discuss in the next chapter.

In concluding this chapter, let's look in more detail at several useful herbs:

Buckthorne (*Rhamnus frangula*)
Part used: bark of a bush dried for more than a year.
Properties: laxative, non-irritating in small doses, stimulates the secretions of the gall bladder, vermifuge, aids formation of scar tissue.
Indications: spasmodic constipation (safe for pregnant women), biliary insufficiency, obesity, cellulite, circulatory complaints and intestinal parasites.
Decoction followed by maceration: 2 teaspoons of bark in 150g of water, to drink in the evenings.

Fluid extract: 1 to 2g per day.
Tincture: 15 to 20 drops, 3 times a day.

Dandelion (*Taraxacum dens leonis*)
Part used: roots, leaves, buds.
Properties: bitter tonic, aperitif, hepato-biliary drainer, decongestant, blood depurative, diuretic.
Indications: colitis, hepatic insufficiency and congestion, lithiasis, hypercholesterolemia, hepatic dermatoses (such as eczema and boils), rheumatism, renal infections, constipation, haemorrhoids, obesity, cellulite. For certain authors, dandelion has an anti-cancer action!
Tincture: 15 to 20 drops, 2 to 3 times a day.

Salad cure during the dandelion season, without throwing away the buds! In *homoeopathy*, *Taraxacum* is a draining remedy particularly indicated in a 'furred tongue' condition. It is also a plant well known in *Chinese medicine*. Among its indications is chronic pelvic inflammation and mastitis.

Celandine (*Chelidonium majus*)
Part used: roots and leaves.
Properties: anti-spasmodic, hypotensor, increases secretion of bile, anti-cancer (?), coricide (to dissolve external growths, i.e. warts), vermifuge, purgative.
Indications: angina pectoris, arterial hypertension, asthma, gastric and duodenal complaints, hepatic and biliary disorders, syphilis (?), intestinal parasites, gastric cancer. *In external use*: warts, corns (fresh sap, only in this use).
Infusion: 15g per litre, 3 times a day.
Tincture: 2 to 5g per day.

CAUTION: *celandine taken orally is very toxic. Its use is therefore not advisable in self-medication.*

ꙮ 14 ꙮ

Cancer

Cancer – that dreaded enigma. It is true that cancer, along with cardio-vascular maladies, is one of today's most fatal diseases, and no other disease evokes the same irrational and visceral fear; no other illness so isolates the victims as if they were our modern-day plague carriers. Because of this reaction, there is an enormous amount of work in the area of support, information, and advice being done by groups of the cancer-stricken and their families (see Useful addresses, page 223).

Mechanisms

Before going into the cancers occurring most often in women (breast, uterus, cervix), let's take a look at the mechanisms at play here, or at least the little of it which is understood.

The mechanism of the 'second liver' has already been discussed (see page 150). However, this is not explanation enough as all benign tumours do not develop into cancer. What characterizes cancer is, on the one hand, the unlimited multiplication of undifferentiated cells, and on the other, the capacity to form colonies in far distant organs and tissues (metastasis). Normally, each cell has a certain programme which dictates the cell's size and work, when to divide, and when to die. This 'intelligence' of the cell is the DNA. The form of the DNA (desoxyribo-nucleic acid) is like that of a twisted rope ladder, each step of which is the carrier of a genetic message. It only takes one link to go awry for the cells to make a mistake and become cancerous. What makes the DNA mutate? Radioactivity (e.g. leukemia in radiologists at the beginning of that specialization), tar (e.g. cigarettes, as has been demonstrated experimentally on rats), certain food colourings or preserving agents, or even a virus?

It has been shown experimentally in chickens that when a certain virus, called oncogenic (that is, which causes cancer), penetrates a cell, it may by substituting its own RNA for that of the cell, mislead the DNA. (The RNA, also a messenger, is one half of the DNA, or the smallest unit from which a filament of DNA can be constituted.) This observation does not yet offer any clear direction in terms of treatment, but it does begin to explain cellular 'intelligence'.

There exists in the organism a system of surveillance of cellular activity and development. This has been demonstrated by experiments on healthy prisoners in whom a melanoma (a particularly virulent form of cancer of the skin) was implanted under the skin. In three weeks, the subjects succeeded in destroying these mutated cells. However, the researchers were not satisfied with this observation and implanted identical cells a second time. To their great surprise, the second time round, the prisoners destroyed the unhealthy cells in *one* week! Their system of surveillance had been put in a 'state of alert' and made even more efficient.

The question which arises from this is: what causes an individual to lose this *immunity*? Certainly, several factors are involved. Those factors which have been recognized include: diet, the environment, psychological and hormonal factors.

(a) *Dietary factors*
These lead us once more to the work of Dr Catherine Kousmine.

Whenever we eat, the fundamental particle involved is the cell, the unit of living matter. For Dr Kousmine, cancer, like multiple sclerosis, is a disease of degeneration in which immunity is increased but inefficient due to a non-receptivity of the cellular wall to the regulatory signals of the body. It is essential to our survival that the membrane of the cell be correctly structured and normally permeable. At the intestinal level, all increases of permeability cause an exaggerated penetration of intestinal content to the interior of the cell. In addition to vital nourishment, however, this content includes toxic substances, bacteria, and viruses. Owing to the fragility of the membrane, it is reconstructed every other day. That is, of all our tissues (cancer included), it is the most rapidly reconstructed. However, in order to be able to construct a normal membrane, our body needs material, that is, adequate food.

Dr Kousmine has long experience in treating the cancer-stricken with dietary changes and polyvitamins. Improvement appears after two months and stabilization after two years. In reading her descriptions of the relapses of persons who return to their former eating habits, one can only be convinced of the validity of her theories (see References)! Another interesting group doing work on diet and cancer is that of Simoneton on the radiation of foods (see Chapter 15).

(b) *Factors linked to the environment*

These are often closely related to dietary ones: presence of colouring or conservation agents or other food additives, cyclamates (banned from sale in the United States because of its carcinogenic effect, though not yet in Europe[1]) and saccharine, nitrites, nitrates, and safol. Food can still *become* carcinogenic in undergoing deterioration during storage (e.g. PCB in silos of milk) or during refining or cooking (e.g. the re-use of frying oil).

Other environmental factors include radioactive radiation (you would not choose to live next to a nuclear energy plant!)

[1] One possible explanation: the consumption is not the same. Swiss legislation requires soft drinks to be sweetened with sugar. In the USA, on the other hand, this is done artificially, resulting in a consumption of artificial sweeteners which is clearly higher. Experiments have shown that an adult would have to consume about 200 cubes of cyclamates over a prolonged period before a carcinogenic threat arises. Hardly to be compared with the usual 3 to 4 daily cups to which we might add artificial sweeteners! Unfortunately, the carcinogenic effects of different products are compounded, even if each product is not consumed at a level reputed to be dangerous.

and pollution of the air and water. We are not the only ones who suffer – forests are dying in countries around the world. I also include here the consumption of alcohol and tobacco, which can be harmful also to those who are not themselves direct users.

(c) *Psychological factors*
Researchers have come to realize that people with cancer often present a particular psychological profile whose dominant traits are passivity and a lack of aggression or the will to live. These traits have been found to play a role in cellular 'self-destruction'. Many people with cancer have suffered a serious emotional shock in the months preceding the appearance of cancer: death of a family member or loved one, marriage, divorce, car accident. These psychological trauma have been codified by, among others, the Simonton group who, on the basis of these observations, have devised a method of healing using self-suggestion which is to be used as an adjunct to other cancer treatments. The exercises consist of visualizing the tumour, and then its healing process through whatever treatment is intended (see References).

All physical and psychological shocks provoke a state of *stress* and a secretion of adrenalin. The entire hormonal system (adrenals, hypothalamus, pituitary gland) reacts to this aggression. This mechanism is, of course, necessary to survival, but equally necessary is a time of recovery once the crisis is past. When already in a state of stress, the use of stimulants (cigarettes, alcohol, drugs) is harmful because it exhausts the system.

It is important to add that the effects of stress on the intestinal mucous membrane is to increase its permeability to a large number of toxins found in the blood which are thus absorbed by the system instead of being eliminated in bowel movements. This represents still more of an overload for the liver, even for a 'second liver'.

(d) *Link between hormones and cancer*
It would appear that an abnormal level of hormones accelerates malignancy. In women, we have a well-known example:

the Pill. Even though it has not been proven that it causes cancer, everyone agrees that it aggravates an existing cancer; the term used is 'hormone-dependent cancer'. The link has been shown many a time between the Pill and cancer of the cervix, or hormonal 'treatments' for menopause and cancer of the uterus! (See for this in relation to the use of oestrogen alone and for the cynicism of the pharmaceutical firms, Barbara Seaman's book under References, *Women and the Crisis in Sex Hormones*.)

I hope these explanations have not been too wearying. Let's look now at something more positive: the possible means of prevention, beginning with early detection. Indeed, modern western medicine often does not detect cancer until it is several months or years old and already involves more than a million cells. At this stage, many forms of treatment are no longer effective!

The figure below shows at which stage the different examinations are able to detect a cancerous state: Breast palpation and the Pap smear are the most frequently used examinations of modern western medicine, even though there are other tests enabling earlier detection.

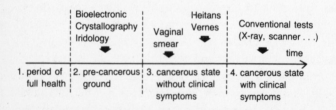

1. *Palpation of breasts* is an examination essential for every woman, and one every woman should be able to do on herself. Having a breast exam once a year, as part of an annual Pap smear, is not sufficient because a cancer of the breast, when given three months to develop, has ample time to metastize in other organs. It is therefore advisable to examine one's breasts once a month, preferably after periods, the moment when the breasts are the least swollen and lumpy.

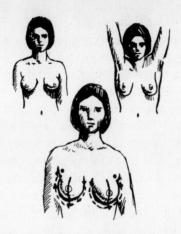

To begin the examination, stand upright in front of a mirror and look carefully at your breasts (see above). Note their shape, any changes since the last examination in their weight, skin texture, or nipples (such as a dimple, as if something is pulling from the interior, or stippled skin, like the peel of an orange). Raising your arms slowly sideways above your head, watch the underside of the breasts, especially how the breasts slide over the ribs (weight and movement).

You can also pull the breasts gently toward the nipple to see if there is any discharge. A milky discharge is normal, even in women who have never breastfed. A discharge of pus or blood is something to discuss with your health care worker.

Still in this position, look for any swollen or tender glands deep in the fold of the underarm or in the hollow of the collarbone. The underarm glands drain the arms and the breasts, in a cleansing, anti-inflammatory, and immunizing action.

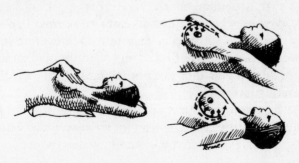

Next, to palpate the breasts, lie down on your back (see above). Doing this in the bath, using soap, isn't a bad idea. To examine your left breast, put your left arm under your head. This spreads the breast over the ribs and moves the pectoral muscle out of the way. With the flat of your fingers of the other hand, examine the breast using a circular pressing movement. Palpation between the thumb and index finger is not advisable because you will run into too many of the breast's 'normal' lumps. This may disquieten you unnecessarily and possibly lead you to abandon a full examination. Do an examination of the entire breast, finishing with the nipple. The upper part of your breast closest to the armpit, generally the most dense part, should be carefully examined. You will vaguely feel your glands as a uniform tissue, grainy and poorly delineated, also, underneath your ribs. What you are looking for is a firmer mass, well-defined, the size of a pea or larger, and independent of the gland.

When you examine your breasts regularly and know them, a new mass is easily distinguished.

Oh yes, I forgot. Afterwards you examine the second breast!

If something appears suspicious, consult a competent person. Three times out of four, detected masses are benign, and for the remaining one, the quicker the mass is detected, the better the prognosis! It is indeed for this reason that breast examinations are so important. The older you become, the more important it is to do this regularly.

2. *Pap smears* can be done less often since cancer of the cervix develops relatively slowly. For most women this means about once a year, depending on the results of the previous examination. Women who have had at least two normal Pap smears in a row can be satisfied with a test once every two years (according to the statistics of the Center of Cytology of Geneva), as long as they are not taking the Pill, which is an aggravating factor.

The Pap smear consists of taking a few cells from around the opening of the cervix, spreading them on a glass slide, and having them examined by a cytology laboratory. A good quantity of cells has to be taken, but not too many because if the layer of cells is too thick it cannot be examined by a microscope.

Pap smears should not be done during menstrual bleeding nor during an infection of the cervix (unless it is a chronic infection and there will not be a better moment) since, at the cellular level, inflammation is still fairly close to a precancerous state. The presence of certain agents, too, such as the virus of condyloma, interferes with results. Another exam, the colposcopy, is done with a huge magnifying glass and a source of light. By putting certain colouring agents on the cervix (Lugol), injured parts can be distinguished from others and it can be determined whether the lesion continues into the cervix or if it is limited.

From the moment a lab report reads 'dysplasia, moderate to marked' (see page 160), it is a good idea to do an examination of the endocervix as well, that is, of the cervical canal (approximately 4cm), and to compare the results in order to decide what to do next.

The detection of cancer of the cervix is the most advanced in the panoply of techniques and has no equal in other tumours which are less easily accessible.

Fortunately, there are other tests which may detect cancer even earlier, although they are not recognized by modern western medicine. I will not be able to describe all of them here, but other authors have already done so (see References).

3. *The Vernes tests*. The Vernes tests are blood tests or, more precisely, tests of the blood serum and its proteins. Using a photometer, the opacity of the serum is studied with different reactive substances, such as acetate of copper. The dosage of muccopolysaccharides is done by orcinol, the calculation of the index of precipitation by euglobulines (see under References). The tests proposed by Vernes beginning in 1936 and improved by his collaborators, including Augusti (Paris), should be considered together for interpretation.

In a diagnosis of cancer, the Vernes tests are not 100 per cent specific for cancer and therefore are not always reliable for diagnosing cancer, but it is in the surveillance and evolution of the diseases that they are irreplaceable. These analyses permit, among other things, to establish (numerically) the extent of inflammation, liver function, and the state of the organism's defence against its disease. They can also be used to select the best moment for surgical intervention and to evaluate the effectiveness of the treatment.

The results of the tests are synthesized on a very 'talkative' curve, the differential curve of Vernes (FRED), which is a kind of electrophoresis of proteins. The difference between the results of the individual and those of the average healthy subject is reported on a table **demonstrating visually (from left to right) hepatic insufficiency, problems with lipids, inflammation, allergies, cancer or, in the case of negative values, a blockage of the reticulo-endothelial system.**

France is little concerned with research and its applications outside of the official line, and after a number of legal difficulties, these tests are no longer available.

Fortunately, other scientists have continued research in a very similar direction and we now have protein profiles (see Reference) at our disposition. These profiles still involve examining several proteins, expressing results in percentages according to the age and sex of the individual. Progress in computers and biochemistry has given us a better understanding of protein dysfunction.

We also have a 'mini-profile' which studies eight proteins both individually and comparatively (IgM, IgG, IgA, C3, seromucoid, transferrin, and albumine) and a more elaborate profile of 15 proteins. In both cases, the results are expressed in comparative percentages and accompanied by a computer synthesized interpretation proposing several possibilities among which only the practitioner can choose, basing the decision on knowledge of the individual concerned. The larger profile is also accompanied by therapeutic suggestions.

Use of this test goes beyond a basic naturopathic gynaecology, but does nonetheless permit us to determine the existence of somatic problems and to detect deep functional problems (problems of 'ground'). The most precise areas of these tests are: inflammation, immune deficiency and response, lack of iron, urinary protein loss (cutaneous or digestive), malnutrition, hepato-cellular insufficiency (including hormonal saturation) and haemolysis (destruction of the red blood cells). There are other kinds of important tests such as *tumour markers*. Only certain tumours are discoverable through tumour markers – notable among those tumours NOT included are breast and lung cancer. Certain progress has been made with tumour markers including CA 15/3 for breast cancer and CA 125 for cancer of the ovary.

Some progress has been made with the discovery of the tumoural brander like the antigen Ca 125, associated with ovarian tumours and the sialic acid.

Let's look then at the three forms of cancer found specifically in women.

(a) *Breast cancer*

I have already talked about detection and tests. Let's assume that the woman has felt a mass, the mammography and the thermography are suspicious. The *surgeons* propose operating along the following lines: first of all, remove the mass. Send it to the pathological lab immediately and wait for the reply before closing the incision. In the event of cancer, they will probably want to remove the breast and at least a few lymph glands under the arm and, finally, scrape a little of the pectoral muscle found under the breast against the ribs. There was a time when they simply removed the breast *and* the pectoral muscle (Halsted operation)!

Where several lymph glands have been invaded by metastases, they will propose local *radiotherapy*. If the metastases have already reached other organs (liver, bone, brain), they will propose *chemotherapy*.

I will not go into more detail on their methods; you will have recognized the lines of modern western medicine, and its literature is vast.

Let's set down the points of controversy.

• *Removal of the entire breast*. Although this is technically rather simple, it is an act which has enormous significance for women. It merits at least a little time for reflection! In addition, the artificial breast (prothesis) that doctors, the medical world and others persuade women to wear is only camouflage for the trauma caused by the loss of a breast. Protheses isolate a woman even more and lead her to believe that the difficult adjustment to the loss of a breast is a personal failure. (See *The Cancer Journals* by Audre Lorde.) The so-called aesthetic operations which implant the protheses are also far from always successful.

- *Removal of lymph glands.* These are an important system of defence for the organism. Those of the underarm drain not only the breast but the arm as well. Thus, when surgeons are too enterprising, women find themselves with arms which are poorly drained, which swell and which have to be re-educated. The loss of the pectoral muscle aggravates this problem still further. Removing lymph glands is a bad practice of surgeons. A monument ought to be raised to the tonsils, adenoids and other appendices which have made surgeons rich; not only are their patients not relieved of their illnesses, their defences are also diminished.

Fortunately, breast cancer surgery has become more and more conservative and it is possible today, if the mass is small and well defined, to remove only the tumour itself and leave the breast. The curettage of the ganglions remains indispensable for surgeons because it gives indications of the spread of the disease and determines the treatment to follow: radiation therapy or chemotherapy. When exposed to cobalt and other rays, the cancerous cells are the first to keel over. Unfortunately, however, neighbouring cells are also affected. In an attempt to limit the damage, the rays are passed through a lead frame, leaving exposed only the part to be radiated. However, rays on the head still cause hair to fall out; on the skin they leave the mark of an old burn, which can itself become cancerous. Chemotherapy is not much less serious. Medication injected into a minor vein injures it. Furthermore, the white blood cells are also attacked by chemotherapy; immunity is thereby diminished. This results in a lowering of resistance to infection which sometimes necessitates isolating the patients.

Clearly, these last two methods tire the organism to such a point that treatments must be spaced out and the patients kept under observation, even hospitalized. Methods evolve continually and today (1993) post-operation therapeutic treatments include 'preventive' radiation and chemotherapy, as soon as a nearby ganglion is affected. When the cancer is already invasive and it is no longer possible to remove it surgically, these methods constitute treatment. Each woman must be informed in detail about the advantages and disadvantages of these methods in order to evaluate for herself the quality of survival these methods bring since they cannot heal.

(b) *Cancer of the uterus*

This generally attacks women older than those with breast cancer. But like breast cancer, cancer of the uterus is more frequent in women who have had few or no children.

The most frequent symptoms are problems with periods, in particular irregular bleeding after menopause. The diagnosis is the result of a rather simple endo-uterine curettage and the examination of the cells removed. Treatment depends on the age and general condition of the woman. When the cancer is in its early stages, or on the contrary inoperable, certain doctors opt for a treatment of progestogens. However, results in these cases are modest and the mechanism unknown.

If the cancer is operable, everyone in modern western medicine agrees on the removal of the uterus. The removal of the ovaries before menopause is more controversial because it causes premature menopause and necessitates replacement hormones. If the cancer is inoperable because it is too advanced (or in a woman too old to take this risk), the most frequently used treatment is the implantation of a small source of radioactive radium in the uterus for a duration of 4 to 6 weeks (a particular form of radiation therapy). General chemotherapy is an option in the most serious cases of cancer.

(c) *Cancer of the cervix*

Like cancer of the breast, cancer of the cervix attacks young women. Thanks, however, to systematic Pap smears, this form of cancer has become much rarer, as it is detected much earlier.

Treatment is, as always, essentially surgical: conization or the removal of the end cone of the cervix. The degree of the amputation (cervix, uterus) depends on the extent of the cancer; after this we come back to the treatments already mentioned: radiation therapy and chemotherapy.

I am aware of having discussed only the generalities of these cancers. There are, of course different kinds of breast cancer and cancer of the uterus. For this kind of information you can turn to modern western medicine, whose classification of these permits a prognosis, a chance of survival.

༄

What are the alternatives?

First of all, dietary changes, giving particular attention to vit-amins (C, A, B complex, E), essential fatty acids (Vitamin F) and trace-elements. There are also numerous less violent treatments than those described above and not recognized by modern western medicine.

I do not have room to talk about all of them here, especially since others have already done it better (see under References, Janet and Lagarde, Adis, Grenoble Group, Forbes).

There are about a dozen reliable anti-cancer remedies, plus several others which can be considered to reinforce immunity, and are therefore useful, even if insufficient in themselves.

Since our experience in this area is limited to a few cases, it is difficult to draw conclusions or give a treatment plan. Let's look instead at what the therapeutic lines might be.

The initial step is to determine the exact diagnosis and extent of the disease, and for this modern western medicine is indeed useful. Next is an evaluation of the woman's tendency to morbidity (pathogenic coefficients of Vernes and Augusti, see page 172), the physical resistance with which she fights against her tumour, and her reserves (immunity coefficient, hepatic index). For example, if her defences have crumbled, it is not advisable to consider an operation. It would be preferable to reinforce these defences first. During this time, anticancer remedies which do not weaken the organism would be used.

In addition to dietary changes, vitamins can be injected in order to compensate rapidly for deficiencies. This is the practice of Dr Catherine Kousmine (see References).

In acute cases, where it is necessary to act quickly and where treatment on an out-patient basis seems difficult, the best collaboration which we have found to date is that of the anthroposophists (Lukas Klinik, Arlesheim, Switzerland – see References).

The anti-cancer remedy of the anthroposophists is fermented European mistletoe (*Viscum album*) or Iscador†. They also work on the 'ground' with the aid of diluted and dynamized minerals and through medicine which is similar to homoeopathy. The basis of the anthroposophic doctrine, broadly speaking, is that when we left the mineral kingdom, we lost a great deal. Minerals, as a living form, have a special force against the exaggerated development of cells. For this reason, minerals (on display and used in therapy) are very important for the anthroposophists. Anthroposophic medicine is a global medicine, centring on three axes: spirit, soul and body. At the clinic of Arlesheim, cancer patients follow different activities: clay modelling (to recapture form), painting, and eurythmics. In addition, anthroposophists truly understand the importance of diet, and serve vegetarian and organic or biodynamic meals.

They are not against all forms of surgery, but prefer it after a treatment of Iscador and a ground treatment. These therapies are continued after the operation. It is necessary first of all to help the organism to build up its immunity system before depriving it of a tumour which serves to maintain a certain equilibrium! The anthroposophists are, on the other hand, generally

opposed to the use of radiation therapy and chemotherapy.
But what do we know about European mistletoe?

European mistletoe (*Viscum album*)
Part used: leaves, young stems of the parasite of the apple tree,
   pear tree, etc.
Properties: vaso-dilator, hypotensor, anti-spasmodic, diuretic,
   decongestant, anti-cancer.
Indications: arterial sclerosis, arterial hypertension, chronic
   nephritis and albuminuria, congestive haemorrhage,
   epilepsy and St Vitus's dance, migraine, asthma, symptoms
   of menopause, cancer.

NO SELF-MEDICATION WITH MISTLETOE IN THIS LAST CASE!

There is a new form of mistletoe available in Germany, due to
the progress of anthroposophic medicine. It is called Vyzorel†
and is used in a perfusion. Its efficiency seems to have increased, including in the presence of metastases.

In the experience of the Women's Health Center, if the
woman does not need to be hospitalized, we would:

(1) talk about diet and outline changes;
(2) discuss other risk factors and attempt to resolve related
    problems (cigarettes, alcohol, the Pill, and stress)

We would look too for a worthy *ally*, one who has experience
with cancer patients and who practices a ground medicine,
that is, centred on the person and not the illness (e.g. naturopaths, homoeopaths) according to the woman's choice. For
the moment, we do not have enough confidence in our treatment alone.

Generally speaking, it is necessary to envisage a year of
primary treatment (Vernes every month to three months), and
5 years of secondary treatment (Vernes every 6 months). This
has been our attitude until now, and although we haven't had
much feedback, we are satisfied.

I will come back to diet in Chapter 15, but I want to explain here what a woman with cancer ought to be particularly attentive to. She should have a diet:

- strictly without sugar
- without white flour or any refined cereal/grain;
- with raw vegetables (depending on the state of the intestine, one can begin with vegetables cooked in water);
- with raw fruit;
- which includes a period cure of vegetable juice;
- without coagulated albumin, such as egg white (on the other hand, raw and fresh egg yolk is good);
- with a little (white) unfermented cheese (processed cheese products are not to be considered 'real' cheese!).

Mother's milk is an excellent food (!) if you happen to know a breastfeeding woman with too much milk.

In short, this is a diet of high radiation (see Chapter 15). It is also important to find a lifestyle which restores your energy. The forest is an excellent environment, according to many, notably the anthroposophers.

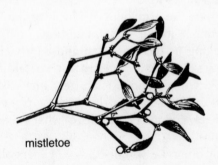

mistletoe

✂ 15 ✂

Diet

In reading the previous chapter, you will have no doubt realized that diet plays a vital role in health and fitness. The functioning of our organism depends entirely on our nourishment.

This is not the end of the matter. There are a multitude of theories claiming to propose healthy or natural diet, which are sometimes contradictory. The Kousmine diet, the raw food diet, the macro-biotic, vegetarian, vegan . . . The result is confusion, disorder, and sometimes even guilt, which doesn't improve one's digestion.

So – what are the principles of a healthy diet? And how can changes be made in our social, emotional and working lives without making us feel on a diet and deprived – something which drives us to deviate, and to a sense of failure?

This subject needs individual attention – difficult to give here. But before discussing the general principles, we can begin with a few concrete examples of what we've encountered in our practice.

The first woman we will discuss is 24 years old. Her arrival in Switzerland, two years ago, constituted a serious uprooting for her and, among other things, a dietary change, which resulted in a gain of 20 pounds.

Her usual diet had been as follows. For breakfast: bread, butter, jam and/or cheese with black tea; at 10 a.m. pastry; at noon (between classes) two to three pastries, sandwiches or pieces of quiche; at 5 p.m. yoghurt with bread and jam, and in the evening, a larger meal with salad, eggs and sausage.

She came to us with complaints of abdominal pains dating back a year; the most serious pain on the right radiating down her leg. In the groin on this side, a painless swelling of the gland was observed. In addition, she was bothered by pains in her breasts which were especially intense at the end of her cycle. She was tired all day long and regained her energy only in the evening. Her eyes ran continuously, and were swollen and sensitive to light.

The situation was clear: her organism was overloaded with sugar and white flour. Animal proteins (the most difficult to digest), eaten in the evening, burdened her system even more and completely overwhelmed her liver. (Remember that in Chinese medicine, problems with the eyes are a reflection of a malfunction of the liver.) She needed to cut down consumption of these foods (sugar, white flour, animal proteins) in favour of vegetables (raw or prepared in a fashion that damages them least – steamed or cooked in a little water, without fat, and seasoned with (cold pressed) oil, lemon, and salt added, fruit and whole grain cereals.

With the aid of a hepato-renal drainer and a hormonal regulator such as raspberry, these dietary changes resulted in an improvement after just one month. The abdominal pains disappeared as did the swelling in her groin. Her skin was clear. She began to lose weight, her eyes no longer ran and she was no longer bothered by light.

You may think that this is an extreme case and that you don't recognize yourself in this example. Good for you!

Let's take the case of an adolescent who thought she ate in a completely 'normal' manner.

She eats white bread and butter, and drinks hot or cold chocolate in the morning; at 10 a.m., a roll; at noon, steak and french fries or fish and potatoes, vegetables, salad, dessert; at 4 p.m., pastries or bread and butter, and in the evening, yoghurt, soup and leftovers from noon.

We won't go into the problems which brought this young woman to us. The dietary problem is the same: there is too much white flour, refined sugar, butter and animal proteins.

Absent from her diet are whole grains, raw vegetables and fruit, and cold pressed oils (eaten uncooked) which contain vitamin E and essential fatty acids, not found elsewhere.

The main problem with the western diet is that we eat too many refined foods and too much animal protein, especially in the evening. By protein, I mean not only meat and sausages, but also dairy products (milk, butter, cheese) and eggs. Often women know that animal protein presents an overload for the organism, and stop eating meat. But they replace it with cheese. This is of no benefit. Only the 'fresh' (non-fermented) cheeses such as fresh goat's cheese are easily digested. The proteins which are the easiest to digest and assimilate are vegetable proteins. These are found in legumes: peas, beans, lentils; all sprouted grains; soya, white, alfalfa; nuts such as walnuts, hazelnuts, almonds; and in whole grain cereals.

The way in which food is prepared is of great importance as overcooking and throwing away cooking water means a loss of vitamins and minerals. When vegetables are cooked in oil or covered with a sauce of milk, cream, or cheese, they are less digestible.

In the preparation of cereals, there is the same problem. When the outer shell is removed in order to whiten it, and when it is ground weeks before it is consumed, vitamins and minerals are lost and only starch is left. Lack of easily digestible protein, of vitamins and minerals, causes deficiencies, and the organism protests!

It is an abberation of 'rich' countries that national diets are both over-rich and lacking in indispensable vitamins and minerals which act as necessary dietary catalysts.

In addition, and this is a problem of city-dwellers, we lead a much too sedentary life. This makes the transformation of highly nutritive foods such as meat (into energy) difficult. In order to 'burn off' a steak, you would have to ride a bicycle to St Cergue (a mountain top near Geneva) and back!

Another dietary problem is the timing and the size of each meal during the day. The 'social meal' is often that of the evening. It is therefore the largest. Unfortunately, it is just at this time that our digestive capacity is at its lowest, even if we stay up late or work nights. Menus are often too complicated: meat, vegetables, a starch with salad and fruit. All of this together presents a very complicated message for the stomach, which, for each of these foods, must secrete a different acid. Raw foods which take longer to digest, get stuck behind cooked food and ferment. The night is a difficult one, with poor sleep or waking towards 2 to 3 a.m. because of indigestion.

In the morning it is difficult to wake up. Your tongue is white, your eyes are perhaps a bit stuck together, and you're not hungry. This is a shame because now is the time when you can take most advantage of the largest quantity and variety of foods. Since you somehow have to get going, you take the first stimulant of the day: coffee. Coffee stimulates intestinal movements; it is for many people the only means of having a bowel movement. But it is also a terrible toxin for the liver; the gall bladder empties and collapses at the arrival of coffee in the stomach! Also, although it provides temporary relief after a big meal, coffee does not facilitate digestion in the long run. It simply retards the sensation of hunger. Though coffee is a prime stimulant, it should be mentioned that this type of stimulation is followed by a drop in energy which is just as spectacular, in the same way white sugar and white flour cause an energy flow like a saw's teeth ∧∧∧∧ , with high peaks and dizzying drops.

A diet based on unrefined foods provides a more even flow of energy ∼∼∼ .

The digestive system can be maltreated for a number of years, but in the long run the effects are felt. The introduction of refined sugar and white flour has caused an increase in diabetes, cardio-vascular diseases, cancer, and dental caries. On this last point, the work of Dr Béguin of La Chaux-de-Fonds (Switzerland) is significant. A study of school-age children revealed a significant correlation between the number of cavities (caries) and the type of diet: either white bread or whole grain, and white sugar or brown or raw sugar.

Dr Béguin shows that *raw* sugar with its richness in minerals encourages healthy teeth. Further, he casts doubt over the improvement supposedly due to flouride. In his study, the children who took it irregularly had better teeth in the end than those who took it regularly! (Is there no justice?) For more details, see References.

Both the work of Dr Béguin and that of Dr Catherine Kousmine demonstrate the link between diet and degenerative illnesses. Particularly interesting is the role diet plays in lowering immunity and resistance to infection, and in the formation of tumours (cysts, fibroids, cancer).

Making a change from a 'western' diet to a strict vegetarian or macrobiotic one results in a marked improvement for the first 3 to 4 years. However, this improvement will only last if the new eating habits are balanced and include sufficient quantities of vegetable proteins. Renewed fatigue and reappearance of illness after 3 to 4 years may lead one to suspect deficiencies and a lack of variety. As you improve your diet, you become more sensitive to deviations from a healthy way of eating. You may react to sugar, coffee, etc. with disagreeable symptoms whereas with a more toxic diet, your organism is too overwhelmed to do more than simply accumulate the toxins.

There are two interesting points which deserve to be emphasized.

First of all, the study of foods which generate acids and bases (see Definitions), proposed by Jackson (see References). Let's remember that our organism, in order to function well, needs a stable pH (measure of acidity) 'mops' (which are bicarbonates and phosphates). Urine and respiration, to a certain extent, rid the body of excess acid or base, but insufficiency of these results in illness.

꙼

Foods generating acids

all meat, including game and fish
nuts

peanuts
beans, dry peas, lentils
refined cereals (white rice, white flour . . .)
sugar
tea, coffee, cacao
all oils and fats (Butter is an acid generator only if it is
   consumed in excessive quantities. In moderate quantity, it is
   neutral.)
cheese
egg white

✌

Foods generating bases

all fruits (fresh and dried), in particular, citrus fruits (lemon,
   orange, grapefruit)
all vegetables (fresh or dried). The leaves of vegetables
   generate more base than the roots.
almonds
cashews
milk (in all forms except cheese)
whole grain flour and products of whole wheat
egg yolk

According to Jackson, the proper balance is ⅘ basis generators
to ⅕ acid generators.

The study of the radiation of foods, according to Simoneton, is
the second most important factor. Everything that lives emits
radiation, and radiation maintains life. All human beings in
good health emit waves from 6,200 to 7,000 angstroms (A°); a
body which emits waves below 6,200° is ill. If the body emits
radiation, it is because it also receives radiation – through
telluric and cosmic waves, waves of the solar spectrum, and the
waves of food products.

Simoneton recognizes four categories of foods, according
to the intensity of radiation that they emit. Foods are

measured for their radiation with the aid of a small apparatus, the *vitalimeter*, which is sensitive to the extra-short waves (that is, lower than 1mm).

(1) *Superior foods (10,000 to 6,500 A°)*
pulp of fruit and fruit juice
organic bread
whole grain cereals, including good homemade pastries.
oily fruits and their oil
almost all raw and steamed vegetables
a few animal products: ham, fish and seafood when fresh and
    raw, very fresh butter, cream and non-fermented cheese,
    freshly laid eggs

(2) *Support foods (6,500 to 3,000 A°)*
fresh milk
pure butter
eggs
honey
sugar
wine
vegetables cooked in boiling water
cooked sea fish

(3) *Inferior foods (less than 3,000 A°)*
cooked meat, offal, sausages
eggs 15 days old
boiled milk
coffee, tea
chocolate
jam
fermented cheese
white bread

(4) *Dead foods (emit no discernible radiation)*
preserved food
margarine
alcohol, liqueurs

refined sugar
baby-food cereals, pasta

Up to this point, the different dietary theories are in agreement and complement one another. There are, however, stricter theories which, though they may suit individual cases, are none the less potentially dangerous.

In Shelton's work on digestible and indigestible associations, for example, he rejects the glucide-lipid association, contrary to what has been said about the rice-bean association, the basic diet for the entire Latin American continent. Macrobiotics theory divides foods into yin and yang, trying to balance roots and tubers with leaves and fruit.

Developing a more refined set of principles can be done only on an individual basis. It is for each person to discover what suits her and what doesn't. One woman's lazy gall bladder may not tolerate onions and cabbage, while for another woman, these are a panacea.

ᴣ

A little advice against constipation

- Drink a lot of fluids,[1] from the moment of getting up, preferably between meals since it is the colon (large intestine) which is in charge of reabsorbing the water and this stimulates it;
- drink lemon juice without sugar before meals;
- decrease the size of the evening meal;
- eat enough fibre (vegetables) and whole grains (with their

[1] Since this is at least the fourth time this piece of advice has been given, the moment has come to add an explanatory note, since even this is the subject of controversy (for example, the macrobiotic supporters are against it). We advise drinking a lot of fluids in order to avoid urinary stasis and to dilute toxins (e.g. antibiotics). However, it is also true that a person with a healthy diet doesn't have to dilute it, and certain people don't seem to need to drink a lot.

outer casing in order to give roughage. Transitionally, take one teaspoon of bran (the outer casing of wheat, sold separately) in a little water 3 times a day.

- Educate your colon by sitting regularly at the same time on the toilet, in the beginning without even having the need to. Take your time, the colon obeys Pavlovian principles quite well!
- Don't use chemical laxatives as they irritate the intestinal mucous membrane. There are, alternatively, quite a few natural methods: prunes or figs, left to soak overnight, or infusions or tinctures of alder buckthorne (*Rhamnus frangula*), flax (*Linum usitatissimum*), dandelion (*Taraxacum*), borage (*Borago off.*), fennel (*Foeniculum vulgare*), senna (*Cassia*), mallow (*Malva sylv.*), etc. The list could go on.

In the case of persistent constipation, it is preferable to use a mechanical aid such as a glycerine suppository which lubricates the bowel movement, or an enema, once or twice a week at the time of dietary changes.

Haemorrhoids are caused by an insufficiency of the deep large veins and a hepatic congestion with a regurgitation into the vena cava. In order to get back up to the heart, blood is borrowed from the superficial veins. These veins, unused to such demands, dilate. (This is the same phenomenon as varicose veins.) Certain factors aggravate a tendency to haemorrhoids: obesity, cellulite, or pregnancy hormones or the Pill. Finally, constipation and the need to push make haemorrhoids bulge out and may even injure them, making them bleed.

The first measure against haemorrhoids is to combat the constipation. Particular attention should be paid to reducing the amount of cooked animal fats, replacing them with vegetable fats. Then everything which improves local circulation is beneficial: cold sitz-baths in the morning, exercise, swimming, and walking. Hot baths are not advisable as they dilate already weak veins. Pain may be relieved by local application of icy witch hazel water.

Constipation may also be improved by the following:

- Trace-elements: Mg (magnesium), Mn (manganese), Co (cobalt), and Li (lithium);
- Herbs in juice form: grape, artichoke, dandelion, bilberry and blackcurrant.

Where a deeper (i.e 'ground') herbal treatment is desired, liver-gall bladder-kidney drainers and herbs with a circulatory action are particularly important. There are numerous possibilities: horse chestnut, witch hazel, cypress, ragwort, pasque-flower, hawthorn, yarrow, goldenseal, bilberry, blackcurrant, shave grass, service tree, hazelnut, broom, chestnut and ruscus.

An efficient formula, including during pregnancy:

tincture of hydrastis
tincture horse chestnut   } aa qsp 90ml
tincture ruscus a.

15 drops, 3 times a day

Most of these herbs have already been discussed in previous chapters, with the exception of the following two.

Horse chestnut (*Aesculus hippocastanum*)
Part used: fruit, bark, leaves.
Properties: vaso-constrictor and vein tonic, blood liquefier, astringent.
Indications: haemorrhoids, varicose veins, liver congestion, problems of menopause, chilblains.
Tincture: 20 to 40 drops a day, before meals, for 10 to 15 days a month.
Bud glycerine macerate: 10 – 20 to 60 drops a day.

In homoeopathy, *Aesculus* is indicated in cases where haemorrhoids bleed little, and where the person has dry mucous membranes and a sensation of having needles in the rectum.

Ruscus (*Ruscus aculeatus*)
Part used: rhizome.
Properties: vaso-constrictor of the vein system (the most

powerful), anti-haemorrhoid, anti-oedema, uric diuretic.

Indications: vein and capillary disease, varicose veins, heavy legs, oedema and leg cramps, haemorrhoids, problems of menopause, painful periods, urinary lithiasis, gout, prevention of post-operative embolism.

Decoction: 60g per litre, 2 to 3 cups a day.

Tincture: 20 to 60 a day.

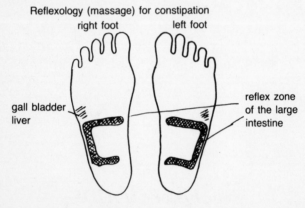

Reflexology (massage) for constipation

Massage the feet, beginning with the right foot, as indicated above. Work round all the zones of the large intestine in a clockwise direction. Massage with both thumbs deeply and stop and spend more time on those zones which are tender or hard. It is important to work on the two angles where the flow may be blocked, especially in the right corner: the gall bladder-liver.

AIDS

As in preceding chapters, we will first take a look at the views of modern western medicine, then at current alternatives.

ॐ

The history of AIDS

The Acquired Immune Deficiency Syndrome, a new sexually transmitted disease, appeared twelve years ago. As its name suggests, it is a disease characterized by a weakened immune system. A person with AIDS dies not of AIDS itself, but of cancer or so-called 'opportunistic infections', diseases which are able to attack the body because the immune system is no longer able to defend itself.

After making its first appearance in Africa, AIDS then turned up in developed countries among gay men, prostitutes and drug addicts. For this reason many heterosexuals believed themselves to be unaffected by this disease. Today the anti-AIDS campaign has spread its message in the gay community, with a resultant drop in infection among homosexuals – and it is largely among heterosexuals that AIDS is spreading! The drama of persons infected by a blood transfusion, both haemophiliacs and others, has only recently been made public. Contamination by intravenous means is the most frequent form of infection, especially in countries where syringes are not sold over the counter. In addition, mother–child contamination is responsible for the infection of 20–40 per cent of babies born to seropositive mothers.

World Health Organisation figures on AIDS are overwhelming: the virus continues to spread inexorably. Black Africa, with 1.75 million cases, remains the continent hardest hit by the virus. In Asia, infection is being transmitted just as quickly while the virus is beginning to ravage Latin America, the Caribbean, the Middle East, North Africa and Central Europe.

Today there is agreement on the means of virus transmission. These include unprotected sexual contact, sharing of needles, contaminated blood and blood products, and mother–child transmission during pregnancy and breastfeeding (see table on page 201). There is a growing progression in the global epidemic among heterosexual women. Perhaps women are more at risk (because of thinner membrane?). Women are often younger than their partners. They find it difficult to impose condoms on their partners even though it is he who more often initiates sexual contact.

The fight against AIDS therefore implies a need to change sexual behaviour: a reduction in the number of partners, the use of both male and female condoms, and the practice of 'safe sex'. The Catholic church continues to oppose the use of condoms, preaching instead marriage and absolute fidelity. Because of its earlier association as 'the gay plague' and because of an unreasoning fear of 'certain death', new marginalized classes are appearing in our societies. In certain countries, such as Morocco and India, seropositive people are locked up. Other countries close their borders, even though systematic testing has not been demonstrated effective. Ostracized, the first victims are in the lowest socio-economic classes. We find ourselves in a situation where millions of people whose immune systems are weakened are ravaged by contagious diseases.

Let's take a look at how the disease progresses, according to three different sources:

(1) After 12 years, in a large group of seropositive homosexual adults in the United States:
  - 25 per cent are still healthy
  - 25 per cent developed symptoms after 10 years, but do not have AIDS
  - 50 per cent have AIDS[1]

(2) At the San Francisco City Clinic, 11 years after seroconversion:
  - 12 per cent are still healthy
  - 36 per cent have minor symptoms
  - 52 per cent have AIDS[2]

(3) Of 562 seropositive homosexuals in San Francisco, after 12½ years of follow-up:
  - 8 per cent have normal CD4 (CD4 is the HIV virus receptor on white blood cells)
  - 31 per cent are asymptomatic or have minor symptoms
  - 69 per cent have AIDS (65 per cent are deceased) (as reported at the AIDS Conference, Berlin, June 1993).

A negative balance sheet but one which still has some surprises:

- the number of seropositive persons who remain healthy
- the length of latency, since fewer than 1 per cent develop AIDS in the first two years after infection
- an 'incubation' which can surpass 12 years, making it impossible to determine whether all those infected will develop the illness
- the number of ill persons presenting all the signs of AIDS without evidence of the presence of the HIV virus.[3]
- Finally, there are seropositive people who have returned to seronegative status, as in the case of Niro Asistente.[4]

Until recently, all research efforts on AIDS have focused on finding the virus responsible for causing the disease. And then one day a storm broke, with great specialists such as Luc Montagnier (who discovered the HIV virus) and Peter Duesberg (who discovered the retro-virus) shaking up medical dogma. The first adopted a critical, although nuanced, approach:

> Research into AIDS suffers from a reductionist approach. Everything happens as if the immune system is progressively killing itself. There are therefore factors which amplify the action of the virus and unfortunately no research programme exists to identify these factors. (Luc Montagnier, *Le Monde*, 25 January, 1992)

The second, Peter Duesberg, contests the link between HIV and AIDS:

> To this day, there has been no controlled epidemiologic study carried out with the purpose of determining whether the HIV virus truly causes AIDS.[5]

AIDS research demonstrates the depth of the debate between different medical approaches. Allopathy still has a penchant for the external causes: everything is the fault of bacteria or a virus. For Duesberg, however, when one looks for a virus, one finishes by finding one, even if it is a weakling such as HIV. (It is because it is such a weakling that its presence is determined only indirectly, through the presence of its antibodies.) In reality, Duesberg maintains, the DNA of each human has for centuries carried between 50 and 100 latent retroviruses, transmitted from generation to generation. In light of this history of retroviruses, why haven't we accorded more importance to the fact that most of the Americans who develop AIDS have been exposed to abnormal health risks: drugs, blood transfusion, use of noxious medication such as AZT, and pre-existing illness such as haemophilia? It has been demonstrated that 95 per cent of contaminated babies were born of drug addict mothers or whose partner was a drug addict or that they had received a transfusion (haemophiliacs for example). Yet their AIDS is attributed to the presence of the HIV virus.

In the past, modern western medicine has vaunted itself as

having conquered tuberculosis through vaccination and antibiotics, although we know that the disappearance of this illness is due more directly to the improvement of economic (and therefore sanitary and nutritional) conditions and that this disappearance had started before the discovery of vaccines and antibiotics. Moreover, tuberculosis is making a comeback. Always a presence where there is poverty, it increases with the rise in poverty that we see in times of economic crisis and debt. Not restricted to so-called Third World countries, the rise in tuberculosis can also be seen among poor people in rich areas such as New York City.

The concept of HIV as sole cause of AIDS pushes research in the direction of anti-viral treatments and vaccines. After 12 years, what has this brought us? The vaccine is difficult to pin down because the virus mutates. It seems there are currently five different versions of HIV. In addition, the eventuality of using a weak and mutating virus for the manufacture of a vaccine can represent an important risk of causing cancer. Despite this, research continues in this direction under the aegis of the World Health Organisation.

With so many unknown factors, where to begin with the origin of this epidemic? First seen in Africa, then in the USA, is it the same virus and, if so, what was its path (Haiti, Cuba)? Or have there been different origins? One other hypothesis[6] attributes the epidemic to widespread smallpox vaccination. There is a correlation between the most vaccinated zones and the countries where AIDS first developed (seven African countries, Brazil and Haiti via the USA), as well as between the vaccination programme and the appearance of the virus. Moreover, the virus of the vaccine was cultivated on the cells of the African green monkey, the origin of the AIDS virus. As a matter of historical precedent, in the 1960s a retrovirus of the same family as AIDS was transmitted from a green monkey to millions of humans by a polio vaccine.[7] The mystery continues, but there is a black-out on discussion of certain hypotheses.

ॐ

What does modern western medicine propose?

So far, modern western medicine has no treatment for AIDS itself. The drugs available are used to extend the life of the patient. Let's look first of all at the inhibitors of cellular division. Currently available remedies are unbelievably expensive and still experimental. Depending on the country, only a part or none of these medications are reimbursed by insurance (in Switzerland AZT and DDI are reimbursed). They have been borrowed from the panoply of cancer-fighting remedies.

> AZT is AIDS by prescription! This substance, zidovudine, interferes with the DNA copying process within the cells, blocking not only the multiplication of the HIV virus, but destroying at the same time all the cells in the process of reproducing, especially the immunity cells.[8]

Unfortunately, we know today that AZT has no positive effect on healthy seropositives, thanks to a French–British study called the 'concord study'. (*Le Monde*, 3 April, 1993).

AZT brings an amelioration in those with AIDS early in treatment, but long-term use seriously lowers overall health and is accompanied by side effects such as anaemia, nausea and vomiting, necessitating the interruption of 'treatment'. During the interruption, general health improves at first but the course of the disease continues. AZT's usefulness remains to be proved. While waiting, many of the ill have swallowed these experimental treatments, some right after seroconversion, others as of the first symptoms or after a fall in DC4, or T cell count, below 350, and many have died while undergoing these treatments.

Added to the effects of AZT are the side effects of antibiotics in the treatment of opportunistic infections. Without these treatments, death is more rapid. (The average survival rate of a person with active AIDS in a rich country is 20 months.) The effect of such immunity enhancers as Interleukin and Interferon has not yet been demonstrated.

Naturopathy, on the other hand, is more interested in attempting to understand why certain people fall ill and others do not. It is therefore interested in endogenous factors, in those characteristics particular to the individual. The fact that the first victims in our country for the most part had in preceding years had numerous infections such as chlamydia, mycoplasma, herpes and other viruses considered much less pathogenic than HIV is completely significant in naturopathy. These infections were contracted during the course of having multiple partners and might have already exhausted the immune system. The consumption of drugs such as cocaine, 'ecstasy' or 'poppers' among homosexuals, the abuse of alcohol, cigarettes, and processed foods are also factors which could explain the loss of cellular intelligence and the exhaustion of the immune response, leaving room for new infections, cancer (such as Kaposi carcoma) and finally death. The fact that AIDS does not express itself at all in the same fashion in Africa as in our country also suggests that it may be necessary to devote more attention to these symptoms and less to the presence of the HIV virus.

The goal in discussing these different theories is not to sow seeds of doubt and insecurity. Duesberg's theories do not mean that it is not necessary to protect oneself (safe sex). On the contrary, it means that Montagnier's theories of cofactors are all the more important. Although reverting to a moralist position of 'who is responsible for the evil?' is not useful, the role of cofactors does mean we need to act on *all* possible factors. Equally importantly, it means that we are not going to blindly submit to the almighty power of a pathogenic virus, leaving us with no escape and no hope.

We know today that stress has a deleterious effect on the immune system by exhausting the cortico-surrenal response used to face stress. Fear also destroys our defences.[9] The equation AIDS = death has certainly increased fear and this fear has shortened the life of more than one person.

A naturopathic treatment therefore begins by a profound

examination into lifestyle, nutrition and habitual ways of dealing with stress. AIDS can be the occasion to become aware and to make profound healthy changes – as was the case for Mark Griffith and others.[10, 21]

But out of respect for the victims of AIDS and those who love them, let's remember in all humility that we still have a way to go until we reach a true understanding and victory over AIDS.

⊰

The alternatives

Diet

Seropositivity, herpes and candidiasis are reminders that our immunity needs better daily support. The human cell needs to be well nourished in order to function effectively. Immune resistance, at the cellular level, relies on the 'waterproofness' of its membrane. Certain elements make this work more difficult, others facilitate it. The appearance of new diseases of an over-stimulated immune system (allergies, self-immune illnesses) or of immunity deficiency is due in large part to the deterioration inherent in overly-refined food. Refined cereals, the use of artificial fats, hydroponics, and on top of everything, the microwave oven, have heavy consequences for our health. When 80 per cent of our daily diet is refined and only 20 per cent is natural, the threshold of tolerance has been largely surpassed.

In short:

- Prioritize living foods, at the height of their maturity and avoid damaging them during preparation. Choose raw or steamed vegetables, cooked or better yet germed or sprouted cereals and legumes (lentils, etc.). *Be Careful: if immunity has already crumbled (CD4<500), avoid raw food!*
- Replace artificial fats (butter, refined oils) with cold-pressed vegetable oils rich in vitamin E and F (linseed,

wheatgerm, evening primrose for making up deficiencies; sunflower, thistle, sesame, walnut, hazelnut and grapestone for daily consumption).
- A basic diet fortified in vitamins A, B and C (for foods rich in vitamin A, see page 13, rich in B, see page 52 and rich in C, tomatoes, rosehip, blackcurrant, cress, chestnut, spinach, cabbage . . .).
- Oligo-elements according to the deficiencies and excesses (as determined through hair analysis)[11] (see annex 3).
- Essential remineralizers: spirulina and other algae; pollen, nettle, shave grass, and alfalfa (eventually in integral suspension of fresh plants), dietary yeasts and mushrooms, oyster powder, etc.

Nourishment of the spirit/energy rebalancing

As numerous authors have demonstrated, depression, fear, and stress lower our immunity. It is impressive to see how beliefs regarding impending death influence the direction of one's present life. An illustration of this is the story of a man locked by accident in a refrigerator truck who died of cold even though the motor was not running. His belief alone killed him. Along the same lines, a number of researchers have been interested in the power of mental healing and in cases of spontaneous healing. Their findings make it impossible to deny the existence of this relationship.[12] Diverse methods exist using the power of the spirit on our health, from auto-suggestion to the Simonton method (see under Cancer on page 167). Bio-energy, yoga and meditation are methods used to regain inner peace and thus health.

The naturopathic methods which take into account the emotional and mental aspects of the person occupy a primary place in the prevention and treatment of AIDS. Examples of these methods are Bach flower remedies, homoeopathy, osteopathy and acupuncture.

Immunity boosters

The following are the immunity boosters of the vegetable world:

In tincture and macerated glycerines:
Echinacea (*Echinacea angustifolia*) (tincture)
Blackcurrant (*Ribes nigrum*) (macerated glycerine)
Sarsaparilla (*Smilax aspera*) (tincture)

In essential oils:
Ravensara (*Ravensara aromatica*)
Eucalyptus (*Eucalyptus polybractea cryptonifer* and *Eucalyptus radiata*)
Thyme (*Thymus vulgaris*)
Melaleuca (*Melaleuca alternifolia* and *Melaleuca quinquinerva (niaoulia)*))
Cinnamon (*Cinnamomum verum*)
Bayleaf (*Laurus nobilis*)
Cohosh (*Caulophyllum inophyllum*)

Echinacea and sarsaparilla have already been addressed in the chapter on herpes and blackcurrant, the major hormonal regulator, in the chapter on painful periods.

Let's look therefore at several new herbs, in the form of essential oils.

Ravensara aromatica ('the guide' according to the profiles of Malhebiau).
Part used: leaves
Properties: antiviral and antibiotic, expectorant, nerve tonic, hypoglycaemic agent, analgesic.
Indications: respiratory afflictions, adenitis, flu, cystitis, diabetes, migraine, parasites, herpes, zona, stress, cramps.
Essential Oil: diluted in 10% in a glycerine alcohol mixture. 2 to 10 drops, 3 times a day.

Eucalyptus globulus ('the renaissance'), or better still
Eucalyptus polycractea cryptonifera as well as
Eucalyptus radiata (fever tree)
Part used: leaves.
Properties: expectorant, bactericide, viricide, antiseptic, hypo-glycaemic agent, anti-inflammatory, febrifuge, stimulant.
Indications: broncho-pulmonary afflictions, flu, cystitis,

diabetes, fever, rheumatism, migraines, parasites, fatigue.

Infusion: 3 to 4 leaves/cup. Decoction 10 minutes. Infusion 10 minutes. 3 to 5 cups a day.

Essential oil: diluted to 10% up to 10 drops, 3 times a day in a little water after meals. (Eucalyptus pol. cry. is contra-indicated for babies, young children, and pregnant women.)

Bayleaf (*Laurus nobilis*)

Part used: leaves, young branches.

Properties: light anti-infection agent, immunostimulant, antispasmodic, lymphatic regulator, nerve tonic, anti-sclerosant, analgesic.

Indications: acne, respiratory and genito-urinary afflictions, flu, arteriosclerosis, adenitis, nevritis anxiety, fear, premature ageing, cancer.

In infusion or essential oils as above.

HIV is found in significant quantities only in blood and vaginal secretions. Contamination therefore can only be through:

(1) unprotected sexual contact, vaginal or anal, sperm in the mouth or other exchange of body fluids;
(2) Transfusion, injection or exposure to contaminated blood or blood products;
(3) Exchange of contaminated needles or syringes;
(4) Mother to child during pregnancy and childbirth.

HIV CANNOT be transmitted by sharing the same school, the same office or even the same plate. The virus does not have the same laws of contamination as most other infectious agents who propagate much more easily, including through the air.

Safe practices

Massage

Masturbation

Kisses, even deep

Kissing and licking the body (except anal and genital mucous membranes)

Rubbing bodies together
Using unshared instruments

Less safe practices
Oral sex on a man (fellatio) or on a woman (cunnilingus)
Vaginal or anal sexual intercourse with a condom (risk of tearing)

Unsafe practices
Unprotected vaginal or anal sexual intercourse (even if there is no ejaculation)
All practices causing bleeding, trauma to tissue followed by unprotected contact, such as the sharing of instruments.

References

1. 'Natural History and Current Therapy', Kenneth M. Mayer, *AIDS and the Health Care System*, Lawrence O. Gostin (Ed.), Yale University Press, New Haven, 1990, pp 21–31.
2. *Pour en decoudre avec: la maladie, les soins, la prévention* . . . , Dialogai and Aide Suisse contre le SIDA, Geneva, April 1992.
3. *The Lancet*, January 29, 1992; WHO communication, Bulletin de l'Office federal de la sante publique, no. 9, Switzerland, March 15, 1993.
4. *Why I Survived AIDS*, Niro Asistente, Simon and Schuster/ Fireside, New York, 1989.
5. 'AIDS Epidemiology: Inconsistencies with Human Immuno-deficiency Virus and with Infectious Diseases.' Proc. Nat. Acad. Sci. USA. Vol. 83, Feb. 1991, pp. 1575–1579.
6. 'Rôle des vaccinations dans la transmission et le déclanchement du SIDA', *Médecines nouvelles*, Paris, September 1987.
7. *L'homéopathie au chevet de la medecine?* Dr. Francois Choffat, Editions Cerf, Paris, 1993.
8. 'SIDA: y a-t-il un scientifique dans la salle?' Comments by Peter Duesberg, collected by Olivier Clerc for Le Lien Santé, June 1992.
9. *Quantum Healing Exploring the Frontiers of Mind/Body Medicine*, Dr. Deepak Chopra, Bantam, New York, 1989.
10. *Rethinking AIDS*, Mark Griffiths, 2040 Polk Street, Suite 321, San Francisco CA 94109 USA.

11. *Equilibre psychobiologique et oligoaliments*, C.C. Pfeifer and P. Gonthier, (Eds.), Equilibre aujourd'hui, Flers, France, 1988.

12. *Alors survient la maladie*, SIRIM, Société Internationale de Recherche Interdisciplinaire sur la Maladie, Ed. Empirika, Saint Erme, 1983.

13. *Etude et prescription de la Medecine Aromatique*, 2 vol. Philippe Mailhebiau, College d'aromatherapie, ZAP du Lattay, Andouille, France, 1992.

14. *SIDA, paroles intimes et nouvelles donnes*, Barbara Pralong, Juliane Robert Grandpierre and Andreas Zulian, Les editions I.E.S., Geneva, 1992.

15. *Le SIDA, guide du praticien*, Dr. Bernard Hirschel, Editions Medecine et Hygiene, Geneva, 1991.

16. *Women and HIV/AIDS, an International Resource Book*, Marge Berer and Sunanda Ray, Pandora Press, London, 1993.

17. *Overcoming AIDS*, Ann Wigmore Foundation, 196 Common-wealth Avenue, Boston MA 02116 USA.

18. *You Can Heal Your Life*, Louise Hay, Hay House, Santa Monica, CA, 1984.

19. *AIDS: The Ultimate Challenge*, Elisabeth Kubler Ross, MacMillan, New York, 1987.

20. *Sauvez votre corps*, Dr. Catherine Kousmine, Editions Laffont, Paris, 1987.

21. *Roger's Recovery From AIDS*, Bob Owen, Davar Publishing, P.O. Box 6310, Malibu CA 90265, 1987.

❧ *Appendix 1* ❧

Definitions

Acuminatum condylomas Warts formed through a local proliferation of the mucous membrane. Of viral origin, they can be found on the vulva, vagina, cervix, perineum, anus or penis.

Acute illness Illness which begins in a sudden violent manner, manifesting itself by inflammatory and infections symptoms.

Adenitis Inflammation of the lymphatic ganglions.

Aerophagia Excess swallowing of air.

Alcohol distillation Maceration of fresh herbs in alcohol. It can be more diluted than a tincture.

Alkaline (or *base*) Chemical compound correlative of acid. A base neutralizes an acid, an acid neutralizes a base.

Amenorrhea Absence of periods.

Analgesic. Medication diminishing the sensation of pain. Also called *antalgic*.

Angina pectoris Syndrome characterized by spasmodic pains in the thoracic region, radiating into the left arm. Almost always due to arteriosclerosis of the coronary arteries or to spasms of these arteries.

Antalgic Remedy or circumstance which results in the relief of pain.

Antibodies The organism's defence agents, whose role is to bind, dissolve and neutralize microbes and toxins. Production of antibodies is stimulated by the presence of antigens, although certain antibodies exist spontaneously in blood serum.

Antigens Substances not recognized as being part of the body (microbes, virus, toxins, etc.) which stimulate the production of antibodies.

Ascaris Genus of round body worms.

Astringent Agent which contracts tissue.

Base See *Alkaline*.

Biliary lithiasis Formation of calculus (stones) in the gall bladder.

'Brake' Remedy capable of braking a hormonal hypersecretion, probably by feedback action (see chapter 5 on amenorrhea).

Buds Buds have the same properties as the plant, but in a more concentrated form. The active principles of buds are best rendered active in an alcohol/glycerine macerate. The first decimal of dilution is used. Preservation of glycerine macerate is the same as that of tinctures.

Calmative Agent with mild sedative or tranquillizing effect.

Carcinoma in situ Final stage before an invasive cancer, or definitive precancerous state. This may be contrasted with dysplasias, where the evolution to cancer is possible, but not a certainty. Here, the entire height of the epithelium is reached, including the surface (see page 160).

Catalyzer Element which, even in very weak quantities, determines modifications in the milieu where it is found, without being itself chemically modified.

Cholecystitis Acute or chronic inflammation of the gall bladder.

Chronic illness Illness which lasts with decreasing and increasing severity. Episodes are less violent than in acute illness. Chronic illness involves the decreased capacity of certain bodily functions and results in a fragile system on which more acute attacks recur periodically.

Cortico-adrenal Tissue of the adrenal gland which secretes about 30 hormones, including aldosteron (diuretic hormones), oestrogens and cortisone (anti-inflammatory and anti-allergy hormone).

Decoction A decoction is obtained by boiling the roots, stems or bark of herbs for 5 to 10 minutes in a covered pot (preferably one of enamel). Decoctions should not be sweetened before drinking.

Depurative Agent which cleanses and purifies the system, especially the blood.

Diuretic Agent increasing urine flow.

Drainer Agent aiding elimination of all wastes, toxins, collection of liquid or other deposits.

Dysmenorrhea Difficult and painful menstruation.

Dysplasia Abnormal cellular development. Dysplasia is divided into three stages: light, moderate and marked. Malignant transformation possible, but not certain. Spontaneous regression possible.

Dystony Disordered muscle tone.

Ectropion The word is used here to refer to an overflow of endo-cervical mucous membrane on to the surface of the cervix. This mucous being more fragile and less able to tolerate the irritations of the vaginal milieu, it is often inflamed, and may even haemorrhage. An ectropion may be due to pregnancy, abortion, or oral contraceptives. It can be sustained by a local irritation.

Electrophoresis Blood test in which blood serum is placed in tubes with different pHs and submitted to a magnetic field, permitting the separation and study of the proteins.

Emmenagogue Agent provoking and regularizing menstrual periods.

Endometriosis Condition in which tissue normally lining the uterus (endometrium) is found in other parts of the body.

Endometritis Acute or chronic infection of the uterus involving primarily the endometrium.

Endometrium Mucous membrane which lines the uterine cavity.

Enema A flushing out, here of the large intestine, using less than a litre of liquid (for example, an infusion of camomile, salt water (at 9gr per cent, like body fluids), or glycerine), which is placed in a jug held 60cm above the body and introduced into the anus through a rubber hose. Lie first on your left side, then on your back, then on your right side. The liquid is held inside about 15 minutes, then evacuated. Enemas may be used in the first months of major dietary changes or before fasting to avoid the excessive passage of toxins through the intestinal wall and the resultant headaches. May also be used in congested states.

Enterocolitis Simultaneous inflammation of the small intestine and colon.

Epidermoid metaplasia Transformation of the epithelium (layer of covering mucus), normally not corneum, into an epithelium which resembles skin. In general, this happens as a response to a chronic irritation of the mucus and is a completely normal means of defence.

Essential oils Aromatic essences are the oily aromatic substances which can be extracted from certain herbs through distillation, infusion, or simple expression. Essences dissolve in oil or in alcohol. Essences which are volatile can be preserved in coloured glass bottles up to one year (see also 'principles of use', Appendix 2).

External use To be applied to the skin.

Febrifuge Agent combatting fever.

Glycerine macerate See under buds.

Ground The body's basic state of health, including individual tendencies to particular illnesses.

Hemostatic Agent which stops bleeding.

Hepatism Term designating the collection of symptoms marking chronic liver disorders: insufficiency, congestion, etc.

Hypercholesterolemia Excess of cholesterol in the blood, a factor favouring cardio-vascular diseases. Cholesterol is a product of the breaking down of the fats involved in the production of sex hormones.

Hypophysis Pituitary gland.

Imitate a cycle Taking oestrogen-like herbs in the first half of the cycle and progesterone-like ones in the second half, interrupting during bleeding. This treatment is repeated for several cycles with the aim of hormonal regulation (to correct conditions such as amenorrhea, sterility, endometriosis, etc.).

Infusion Infusions are obtained by pouring boiling water on to the leaves of dry or fresh plants. A pinch corresponds to 2 to 3g, a dessertspoon to 5g, a tablespoon to 10g and a fistful to 30 to 40g per litre of water.

Internal use To be taken orally or via the anus or vagina. Absorption takes place through a mucous membrane.

Leucoplakia Whitish spot on a mucous membrane (here the cervix) which may be of varied origin. A layer of keratine is formed and comes off in patches.

Leukorrhea White vaginal discharge.

Lithiasis Tendency to form stones.

Lutein Former name for progesterone.

Lymphatic system One of the systems of defence, the 'sanitation department' of the organism, it includes the lymphs, their channels and glands.

Metrorrhagia Uterine haemorrhage occurring outside of menstrual periods.

Nephritis Acute or chronic inflammation of the kidneys.

Neuro-vegetative system Nervous system independent of central nervous system and situated in the ganglion chains which run along both sides of the spine. Functions by a very complex reflex system with two secretions with opposite actions, adrenaline with sympathetic action and acetyl-choline with parasympathetic action.

- *Sympathetic action* Accelerates the heart, contracts the veins, raises arterial tension and sugar in the blood, inhibits bronchial and intestinal muscles.

- *Parasympathetic action* Dilates arteries and capillaries, reinforces contractions of the digestive tubes, sets off contractions and hypersecretion of bronchial tubes.

Ovaritis Inflammation of the ovary.

Oxyuris Family name for human threadworm.

Parakeratosis Change in the appearance of the epithelium which decreases in thickness and forms a 'keratine' (horny layer). Not considered precancerous.

Parasympathetic See under Neuro-vegetative system.

Peritonitis Acute or chronic inflammation of the peritoneum (outer casing of the intestines).

Phytotherapy Herbal medicine.

Plethora Old term meaning over-abundance of blood and

'humour' in the organism. It is attended by a feeling of tension in the head, a florid complexion, and tight and shiny skin.

Polyps of the cervix Protruding growth from a mucous membrane on the cervix or in the uterus and protruding from the cervix. There is often an associated dermoid metaplasia, and the surface of the polyp can ulcerate or bleed (contact bleeding). Malignant transformation very rare.

Progesterone-like Imitates progesterone. Includes herbs such as yarrow, chaste tree, gromwell, tansy, meadowsweet and stoneseed.

Rate of sediment Test performed on blood placed in a tube, examining the quantity of sediment after a certain period of time.

Retroflexion Position of the uterus where it is tipped back against the colon (anteverted) (see below).

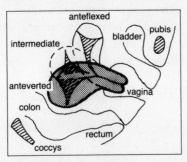

Revulsive Agent which draws blood from one part to another.

Safol Preponderant liquid constituent of sassafras oil.

Salpingitis Acute or chronic inflammation of Fallopian tubes.

Steroid-like Imitates the group of genital and cortico-adrenal hormones. Includes herbs such as blackcurrant, sage, raspberry, rose hip and bramble.

Sudorific Agent promoting perspiration.

Syndrome Set of symptoms occurring at the same time. (Generally employed in place of 'disease' when there is a doubt about the causes or the connections of these symptoms.)

Tincture Tinctures are macerations of fresh or dry herbs in alcohol or other appropriate liquid. They are the basic materials of homoeopathy. In a bottle of coloured glass and protected from heat, they can be kept for one year.

Tonic Stimulant which activates and reconstitutes the forces of the organism, increasing vital resistance.

Trace-element Trace-elements are metals suspended in a liquid. Their action is not quantitative, but qualitative. They are catalysers in the reactions of the organism. Trace-elements are in a week and dynamized dilution. For best absorption, place under the tongue in the morning before eating.

Urinary lithiasis Formation of crystals (calculus) in the kidney.

Vasomotor Relating to the dilation and contraction of veins.

Vermifuge Agent causing expulsion of intestinal worms.

Vulnerary Agent which aids in scar formation.

Zone of junction Intermediary zone between the glandular zone (endocervical) and non-glandular (exo-cervical), forming a white border which does not collect iodine.

Zone of regeneration Following an attack on the cervical mucous membrane, there is a reconstruction of the mucus with normal cells.

✂ *Appendix 2* ✂

The Use of Essential Oils and Tinctures: a Few Principles

On the skin

Although tinctures such as calendula can be used undiluted on the skin, it is better to dilute them in a little water. The dilution may range from a few drops in a little water up to a teaspoon of tincture per cup of water.

Essential oils too can be used in concentrated form, but again it is better to dilute them in oil or glycerine. For example,

in sweet almond oil;
in a cream:
cetylic alcohol   4g
lanoline   10g
white vaseline   86g

The essential oils are added in a quantity of up to 15 per cent. In other words, 15g of a total 100g.

in a bath.

ぞ

On a mucous membrane
(vaginal use, for example)

For use on a mucous membrane, tinctures are used *only* in diluted form. The proportions may range from ½ teaspoon to a litre of liquid to 1 spoonful per ½ litre.

Essential oils are not used in undiluted form on mucous membranes because they burn. Since they cannot be diluted in water, we have to use something like the following:

An oil:

sweet almond oil	60g
wheat germ oil	20g
essential oils	2g maximum

In cream form:

hydrophile unguent	100g
1 per thousand	
castor oil	5g
essential oils	0.5g to 1g of each
(2 to 3 herbs)	
camomile oil	2.5g

In ovule (suppository) form:

EO x	
EO y	1 drop of each
EO z	
tincture calendula	
tincture comfrey	aa 0.03
green clay	0.075g
vitamin E	0.05g
excipient	qsp 1 ovule of 5g

One ovule each evening.

ॐ

Orally

Tinctures to be taken orally can be diluted in a little water. Essential oils, however, may not – they do not dissolve and can burn the stomach. Even honey cannot be recommended as an excipient. Instead, glycerine or alcohol should be used.

For example:

essential oil	6g
alcohol 94%	50g
glycerine 98%	20g

10 to 25 drops, 2 to 3 times a day, depending on the acuteness of the ailment and on individual tendencies.

Essential oils can also be diluted in hydrolate of soya, which appears to form a finer emulsion and increase tolerance. When using hydrolate of soya, the proportion of essential oils can range from 10 to 20 per cent of the solution.

Tinctures are taken before meals, essential oils after meals, in a little water.

ॐ

Enemas

For use in enemas, essential oils can be mixed in the following fashion:

EO	5g
sweet almond oil	50g
oil of grapeseed, wheat germ, or paraffin	50g

Each dose should contain 10g, diluted in 25 or 33cc of one of the oils used in the preparation.

❧

Dosage for children

(fractions are those of an adult dose)

	Infusion Decoction	Essences Tinctures
from 1 to 3 years	⅙	¹⁄₂₀
3 to 7 years	¼ to ⅓	⅙
7 to 12 years	⅓ to ½	¼ to ⅓
12 to 20 years	⅓	½ to ⅔

When using tinctures, you can also follow the rule of thumb of 1 drop per kilo of the child's weight per dose.

❧

Dosage for women

All of the doses mentioned in this book are average doses. To tailor them to the individual, the weight of the woman and her diet have to be taken into consideration. A woman with a 'clean' diet, who doesn't smoke, will respond to a smaller dose than will a woman with a heavy diet or a woman who smokes a lot.

✥ Appendix 3 ✥

The Diathesis in the
Use of Trace-Elements

The trace-elements discussed in this book are not to be thought of as having a quantitative effect, taken to counteract a deficiency. Rather, they act as a catalyser whose presence helps regularize cellular exchange and physio-chemical metabolism.

A diathesis describes an intermediary state between health and illness. In other words, there is a progressive dysfunction or disequilibrium. These diatheses are not static, and each one of us moves between diatheses as we move between health and illness or between illness and health.

The classification of diatheses, like all typologies, is a bit arbitrary. The vocabulary used, including that describing behaviour, does not distinguish between women and men. Menstrual problems are simply added to other symptoms which are improved by a particular trace-element. Similarly, the descriptions do not take into consideration the fact that certain words may not mean the same thing when applied to women as they do when applied to men – 'aggressiveness', for example. Unfortunately, we still lack a feminist medical terminology and a typology devised by us (although some women find certain indications in astrology, to cite one example).

In the meantime, these descriptions continue to provide information, as here where it is not advisable to select trace-elements based only on one or two of the symptoms or illnesses. Behaviour is always the most significant factor in the choice of a trace-element.

(1) *Allergic (Mn or manganese)*

The allergic woman wakes up tired and gains energy only by engaging in some activity. In the evenings she becomes a little euphoric and has difficulty falling asleep. She can also be described as forgetful, optimistic and aggressive.

The symptoms to which she may be susceptible include: migraine, eczema, hives, asthma, colds, hypotension, angina pectoris, arthritis, liver problems related to migraines or fatigue, colitis, gout, fibroids, painful periods and thyroid problems.

Mn can be associated with sulphur for liver problems and with iodine for thyroid problems.

(2) *Lypostenic (Mn-Cu, manganese-copper)*

Also called athro-tuberculosis, this diathesis is especially characterized by fatigue. The more the day wears on, the more a woman in this diathesis becomes tired. Her fatigue, however, yields easily to rest. In fact, she needs a lot of sleep and vacation time. She is pessimistic and cautious.

She is bothered by a sensitive respiratory system (colds, sinusitis, tuberculosis), by lymphatic reactions, duodenal problems, light cystitis, a tendency to hypothyroidism, feeling the cold acutely, painful periods, anaemia, looseness in ligaments, signs of arthritis, bronchial asthma and headaches.

(3) *Dystonic (Mn-Co, manganese-cobalt)*

Also called neuro-arthritic, this diathesis most often evolves out of the allergic diathesis. A woman in the dystonic diathesis is tired all day long with drops in energy before meals and around 5 p.m. This fatigue is accompanied by heaviness in the legs. The dystonic woman is forgetful, anxious, emotional, or depressed. Sleep is mediocre. She is bothered by neuro-vegetative dystonies, spasms, swelling of the extremities, circulatory problems, digestive problems (stomach aches, bloatedness, spasmodic colitis), changes in blood pressure, pre-menopausal and menopausal problems, haemorrhoids, and pelvic congestion.

Improvement is brought about by prolonged treatment (10 to 16 weeks) of Mn-Co.

(4) *Anergic (Cu-Au-Ag, copper-gold-silver)*

The anergic woman is characterized by swings between euphoria and aggressiveness. She seems a little disgusted by life. She is the prime example of someone overstrained by modern times. Her sleep is irregular with insomnia and nightmare. She is bothered by chronic infections, sore throats, cystitis, inexplicable fever, acute articular rheumatism and viral infections.

The action of Cu-Au-Ag is always ephemeral. It provides support for an antibiotic treatment, and is particularly effective in difficult convalescences after a long infectious illness.

Although Cu-Au-Ag is taken over a short period of time, doses are tapered off gradually. Three times a week for two weeks, twice a week for one week, once a week for one week, and stop.

(5) *Syndrome of maladaption (Zn-Cu or Zn-Ni-Co, zinc-copper or zinc-nickel-cobalt)*

This is the diathesis of functional endocrinological problems or of stress. Fatigue is periodic and ephemeral. Irregular drops in energy are accompanied by depression. Symptoms are all dysfunctions which are endocrinological, pituitary (menopause), adrenal or pancreatic (colitis, bloatedness, prediabetes), sexual indifference, loss of hair and problems with fingernails.

This diathesis often comes 'on top' of another diathesis and is always transitory. It is a diathesis of transition. These trace-elements may be taken in order to make another diathesis appear.

These associations of trace-elements are contra-indicated in cancer and tuberculosis.

We might mention that there are other trace-elements (such as lithium, aluminium, sulphur and bismuth) which can be useful in other ailments. For more information, see References.

✣ *Appendix 4* ✣

Table of Brand and Generic Drug Names

American	Swiss	Generic
Amoxicillin	Clamoxyl	amoxycillin
Ampicillin	Penbritin	ampicillin
Cleocin HCl	Dalacine	clindamycine
Danocrine	Danatrol	danazol
Erythromycin	Erythromycine	erythromycine
	Fasigyne	imidazole
	Gynosterosan	chloroquinaldol
	Lactoferment	cultura lactobacill.
Fungizone	Amphocycline	amphotericine
Monistat	Monistat	
Motrin	Motrin	ibuprofen
Mycostatin	Mycostatine	nystatine
Nupercainal	Nupercainal	hydrochloride of cinchocaine
Pergonal	Pergonal	FSH + LH
Ponstel	Ponstan	mefenamic
Premarin	Premarin	conjugated equine oestrogens
Sultrin	Sultrin	sulphathiazole
Terramycin	Terramycine	oxytetracycline
	Tiberal	ornidazole
Trobicin	Trobicin	spectinomycin
Viranol	Vagoclyss	lactic acid
Vibramycin	Vibramycine	doxycycline

References

(1) Books by women

The Cancer Journals, Audre Lorde, Spinsters' Ink, New York, 1979.

The Childbearing Year, a wise woman herbal, Susan Weed, Ash Tree Publishing, Woodstock, N.Y., 1985.

Examen gynécologique et infection, Des femmes du Centre femmes, Genève, September 1976.

'Herpease', Kristine Kellehouse and Chavola Esparza, *The Hot Flash*, quarterly, Women's Health Service, Sante Fe, New Mexico.

Healing Wise, a wise woman herbal, Susan Weed, Ash Tree Publishing, Woodstock, N.Y., 1989.

How to Stay Out of the Gynecologist's Office, Federation of Feminist Women's Health Centers, with illustrations by Susan Gage, Peace Press, Culver City, California, 1981.

Lesbian Health Matters, Santa Cruz Women's Health Collective, 1979.

A Modern Herbal, 2 vols, M. Grieve, Dover, New York, 1971.

Newsletter and *Broadsheets* published by the Women's Health Information Centre (see under Useful addresses).

A New View of Woman's Body, Federation of Feminist Women's Health Centers, with illustrations by Susan Gage, Simon & Schuster, New York, 1981.

Our Bodies, Ourselves, Boston Women's Health Book Collective, Simon & Schuster, New York, revised edition.

'The use of herbal birth control among Indian women in North America', article by Barbara Kean in a Boston Women's Health Book Collective Information Package, 1977.

Witches Heal – Lesbian Herbal Self-sufficiency, Billie Potts, Hecuba's Daughters, Bearsville, New York, 1981.

Witches, Midwives and Nurses, Barbara Ehrenreich and Deirdre

219

English, Glass Mountain Pamphlets, Oyster Bay, New York, 1973.

Women and the Crisis in Sex Hormones, B. and G. Seaman, Bantam Books, New York, 1978.

Womenwise, women and health quarterly published by the New Hampshire Feminist Health Center, 38 South Main Street, Concord, New Hampshire, 03301 USA.

(2) *Natural healing and diet*

Aliments naturels, dents saines, Max-Henri Béguin, Editions de l'Etoile, La Chaux de Fonds, Switzerland, 1979.

The Dictionary of Minerals – the Complete Guide to Minerals and Mineral Therapy, Leonard Mervyn, Thorsons, Wellingborough, 1984.

The Dictionary of Vitamins – the Complete Guide to Vitamins and Vitamin Therapy, Leonard Mervyn, Thorsons, Wellingborough, 1984.

Diet for a Small Planet, Frances Moore Lappé, Ballantine Books, New York, 3rd edn 1983.

Guide de radiesthésie, Michel Moine, Stock, Paris, 1983.

Guide des plantes médicinales, P. Schauenberg and F. Paris, Delachaux et Niestlé, Neuchâtel-Paris, 1977.

Homoeopathic Green Medicine, A.C.G. Ross, Thorsons, Wellingborough, 1978.

How to be Always Well, Robert G. Jackson.

The Illustrated Herbal Handbook, Juliette de Bairacli Levy, Faber, London, 1982.

Indian Herbalogy in North America, Alma R. Hutchens, Merco, Windsor, Ontario, 1973.

La médecine par les plantes, Jean-Marie Pelt, Fayard, Paris, 1981.

Laurel's Kitchen, L. Robertson, C. Flinders, B. Godrey, Bantam Books, New York, 1976.

Les trajets de l'énergie, Robert Courbob, Ed., d'Istor, Paris, 1986.

L'Officine, F. Dorvault, Vogot, Paris, 1978.

Mind as Healer, Mind as Slayer, Kenneth R. Pelletier, Allen & Unwin, London, 1977.

Naturopathic Medicine, Roger Newman Turner, Thorsons, Wellingborough, 1984.

Phytothérapie, aromathérapie, traitement des maladies par les fruits, les légumes et les céréales, Dr. J. Valnet, Maloine, Paris, published annually.

Phytothérapie et aromathérapie, J. Valnet, Durrafour, Lapraz. Presse de la Renaissance, Paris, 1979.

La phytothérapie rénovée, Tetau et Mergeret, Maloine, Paris, 1972.

Précis de phytothérapie, H. Leclerc, Masson, Paris, 1976.

Radiation des aliments, André Simoneton, Le Courrier du Livre, Paris, 1971.

La radiesthésie ou le pouvoir du pendule, Tchou, Paris, 1981.

Traité de phytothérapie et d'aromathérapie, 3 vols, M. Girault, Maloine, Paris, 1979.

Vitamines et vitaminothérapie, Dr Claude Binet, Editions Dangles St Jean de Fraye, France, 1981.

(3) *Natural healing and cancer*
The Bristol Diet, Alec Forbes, Century, London, 1984.

Fighting for Our Lives, Kit Mouat, Heretic Books, London, 1984.

A Gentle Way with Cancer, Branda Kidman, Century, London, 1983.

Getting Well Again, Carl Simonton, Stephanie Matthews Simonton, James Creighton, Bantam Books, New York, 1982.

Soyez bien dans votre assiette jusqu'à 80 ans et plus, Dr Catherine Kousmine, Tchou, Paris, 1980.

Le traitement des cancers par les méthodes de Vernes, Dr J. Janet, Editions Bio-mat, Bordeaux.

(4) *Modern western medicine*
Encyclopédie médico-chirugicale, Editions Techniques, Paris.

Les infections, J.C. Pechère, Maloine, Paris, 1979.

'Infections of the urinary tract', Robert H. Rubin, *Scientific American*, 1982.

Obstetrics and Gynecology, R. Benson, Lange, California, 1974.

(5) *Chinese medicine*
A Barefoot Doctor's Manual, Revolutionary Committee on Health of the Hunan Province, Cloudburst, California, 1977.

Chinese Herbal Medicine Richard Hyatt, Thorsons, Wellingborough, 1978.

Do-It-Yourself Shiatsu, Wataru Ohashi, E.P. Dutton, New York, 1976.

La médecine chinoise par les plantes, Dr Wong, Tchou, Paris, 1976.

(6) *Homoeopathy*
The Organon, S. Hahnemann.
Repertory of homeopathic matiera medica, J.T. Kent, B. Jain Publishing, New Delhi, 1972.
Matiera Medica, W. Boericke, B. Jain Publishing, New Delhi, 1978.
La balance tropique, D. Senn, Fond. Cornelius Celcius, Lausanne, 1980.
Tout savoir sur l'homéopathie, Y. Maillé, Favre, Lausanne, Paris, 1986.

(7) *General books on alternative medicine*
The Alternative Health Guide, Brian Inglis and Ruth West, Michael Joseph, London, 1983.
The College of Health Guide to Alternative Medicine, Ruth West, College of Health, 18 Victoria Park Square, London E2 9PF.

Useful Addresses

Principal European women's groups

Belgium
Aimer à Louvain la Neuve, Cour des 3 Fontaines 31, 1348 Louvain la Neuve.

England
Women's Health Information Centre, 52–54 Featherstone St, London EC1.

France
L'Impatient, 9 rue Saulnier, F-75009, Paris.

Netherlands
Vrouwengesondheidscentrum, Obiplein 4, 1094 RB Amsterdam.
Vrouwengesondheidscentrum, Maliesingel 26, 3581 Utrecht.
Women's Global Network for Reproductive Rights, Nieuwe Zijds Voorbulgwal 32, 1012 RZ Amsterdam.

Switzerland
Frauenpraxis Paradies, Paradiesstr. 11, 4102 Binningen (Basel).
Frauengesundheitszentrum, Aarberger gasse 16, 3011 Bern.
Espace Femmes International, 2 rue de la Tammerie, 1227 Carange, Geneva.
Centre Femmes et santé, 21 rue Haute, Colombier 2013
Frauen Ambi, 27 Mattengasse, 8005 Zurich.

Germany
Feministische Frauengesundheitszentrum, Bambergerstrasse 51,
1 Berlin 30.

Organizations in the UK

**These associations keep lists of registered practitioners and maintain a
check on standards.*

*British Homoeopathic Association, 27a Devonshire Street,
London W1
*British Naturopathic and Osteopathic Association, Frazer House,
6 Netherhall Gardens, London NW3.
*Society of Homoeopaths, 101 Sebastian Avenue, Shenfield,
Brentwood, Essex CM15 8PP.
British Society for Nutritional Medicine, c/o Dr Alan Stewart,
Information Officer, 5 Somerhill Road, Hove, Sussex BN3 1RP.
The Herb Society, 34 Boscobel Place, London SW1W 9PE.
Dalston Children's Centre and Alternative Health Group, 112
Greenwood Rd, London E8.
Community Health Foundation, 188–194 Old St, London WC1V
3BP.
Natural Health Network, Chardstock House, Chard, Somerset
TA20 2TL.
*Institute for Complementary Medicine, 21 Portland Place, London
W1N 3AF.
*Anglo-European College of Chiropractic, 13–15 Parkwood Rd,
Bournemouth, Dorset.
Association of Unani and Ayurvedic Practitioners in UK, 36 East
Street, London W1.
National Institute of Medicinal Herbalists, School of Herbal
Medicine, 148 Forest Rd, Tunbridge Wells, Kent.
*National Institute of Medical Herbalists, Hatherley Rd,
Winchester, Hampshire.
*British Acupuncture Association and Register, 34 Alderney St,
London SW1.
Traditional Acupuncture Society, 11 Grange Park, Stratford-on-
Avon, Warwickshire CV37 6XH.
Register of Traditional Chinese Medicine, 7a Thorndean Street,
London SW18.

Bristol Cancer Help Centre, Grove House, Cornwallis Grove, Clifton, Bristol.

Association for New Approaches to Cancer; c/o The Seekers Trust, Addington Park, Maidstone, Kent ME19 5BL.

Cheltenham Cancer Help Centre, 51 Rodney Road, Cheltenham, Glos GL50 1HX.

Holistic Council for Cancer, Runnings Park, Croft Bank, West Malvern, Worcs WR14 4BP.

Cancer Link, 46a Pentonville Road, London N1 9HF. Can put people in touch with local support groups.

Moira Carpenter, 55 Mallard Place, Strawberry Vale, Twickenham, Middlesex. (PMS centre based on alternative medicine).

Health for the New Age, 1a Addison Crescent, London W14 8JP.

Selected groups in the USA

Federation of the Feminist Women's Health Centers, 2460 E. Balfour Avenue, Fullerton, CA 92631.

Berkeley Women's Health Collective, 2908 Ellsworth, Berkeley, CA 94705.

Coalition for the Medical Rights of Women, 433 Turk Street, San Francisco, CA 94117.

Santa Cruz Women's Health Collective, 250 Locust Street, Santa Cruz, CA 95060.

Women's Health Services, 111 East Dale, Colorado Springs, CO 80903.

Emma Goldman's Women's Health Center, 1628 West Belmont Avenue, Chicago, IL 60626.

Emma Goldman Clinic for Women, 227 N. Dubuque, Iowa City, IA 52240.

Boston Women's Health Book Collective, Box 192, West Somerville, MA 01244.

New Hampshire Feminist Health Center, 38 South Main Street, Concord, NH 03301.

Vermont Women's Health Center, 336 North Avenue, Burlington, VT 05401.

The National Women's Health Network, 224 7th St SE, Washington DC 20003.

Women's groups in Canada

Vancouver Women's Health Collective, 1501 W. Broadway, Vancouver, BC.
Centre de santé des femmes du quartier, 16 Est Bd St Joseph, Montréal.

Selected groups in Australia

Leichhardt Women's Community Health Centre, 164 Flood Street, Leichhardt, New South Wales 2040.
Adelaide Women's Community Health Centre, 2 King William Road, NRTH Adelside, 5006.
Liverpool Women's Health Centre, 273 George Street, Liverpool.

Women's group in New Zealand

Hecate Women's Health Collective, P.O. Box 11–675, Wellington.

General Index

Index of Herbs

(English names)